DIAGNOSIS MULTIPLE SCLEROSIS

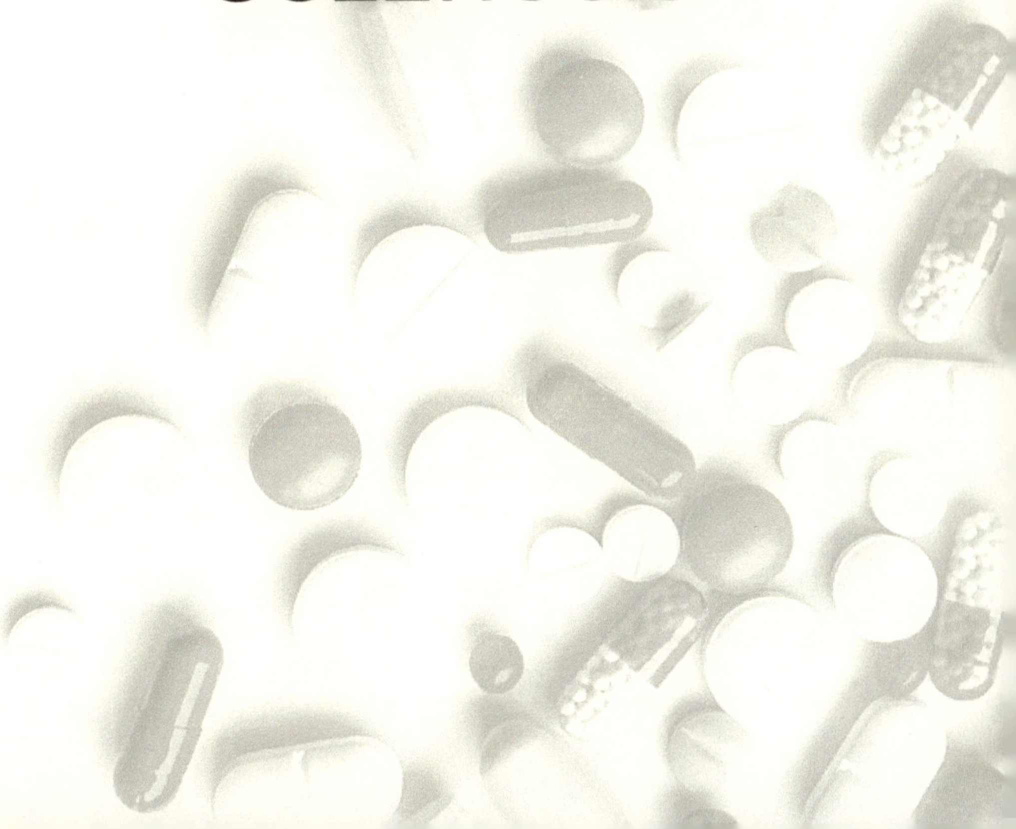

DIAGNOSIS MULTIPLE SCLEROSIS

The Journey Through a Lifelong Health Condition

M C Stuart

978-1-80541-186-4 (paperback)
978-1-80541-187-1 (ebook)

CONTENTS

INTRODUCTION

It is my will that I aim to benefit people, and myself, with a bunch of information that is inspiring and educational and based on my health experiences, encouraging you to learn to live with what life throws at you and keep going with determination. I want people to endure the trials they face, and, like me, to be happy with the journey and take the good with the bad. There are actions I take and some that I avoid, and, given the gravity of my situation, I am keeping it together mostly. The actions I take help me to cope with my health issues and lead to a rewarding life even with my lifelong health condition. Can you think of actions you can take? People may find something in here that benefits them. The best advice is to be actively at work against ill health and live a life free from indisposition. Enjoy the highs and lows with positivity and an eagerness to learn.

My health is under attack by multiple sclerosis (MS) and will keep me under threat, so this is my motivation to action because I want to survive. The damage to my nervous system has been caused by my immune system misbehaving and leaves me with a variety of problems. My immune system has started attacking my nerves at times and the damage may be irreversible. The nerves have a coating that protects them and when this coating gets damaged, it causes me to develop movement and sensory difficulties, especially when I'm in hot weather for too long. It can even affect my cognitive functions which are my psychological types and my behaviour. If the damage persists, it can get to the nerve fibres and even damage them and this damage will mean I lose some control permanently and totally alter my life, so I don't want that to happen.

MS has been a very slow process in my case. I think that sometimes a case can be very aggressive and cause fast deterioration and this is so unfair. Fortunately for me, it is very un-aggressive, and this has given me time to adapt. If untreated, it will damage the actual nerve tissue and that would be bad, so I take it a day at a time, and the best way I deal with things is to think about the current day and not focus on tomorrow. In this way, I can make decisions on personal treatment. Tomorrow is where I will come to but not until I have finished with today. This way, I don't overburden myself with worry. I simply make sure I am always aware of my eyesight, balance and level of fatigue.

If I put my mind to it, who knows what my body is capable of? The process I write about is what I have learned from all the experiences I have been through and what I have gained in understanding what works for me. I want to live and go through all the effects as part of *life*, rather than the alternative.

I do think I can make a difference in my health, otherwise, I don't think I would work as hard on it. I only listen to this belief and want to be living proof of what can be done if a person puts their mind to it. I am going to spend my time working on the solution to my MS problem and following the thread running through this book about living a healthy lifestyle.

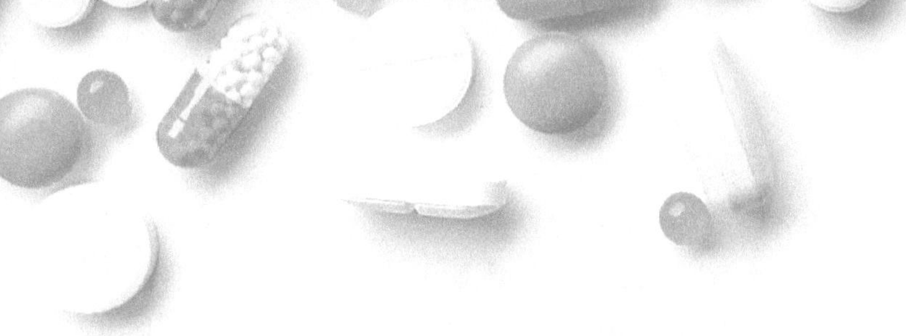

CHAPTER 1

How it all began to take shape

When I was young, I was enjoying life, I was doing whatever I wanted and often stayed out all night partying with friends. Basically, I had no worries. That doesn't mean I had nothing I could worry about, but more that I didn't care much. This situation is never going to last for anyone, but at the time, I didn't realise how shallow and immature I was being. Could it be that I thought life was going to be like this and never change? Was that just naivety? Really, I lacked any understanding of things and treated life as if it was just a big game. This was all pre-MS, and for me, it lasted decades. Thinking back, I see how I was going wrong and how lucky I am that it didn't end up as something worse than a few mishaps. There are some mistakes I made on purpose to see what it was like, and you could say I was out of control for some years.

I kind of turned my life around in my twenties though, but still had dark thoughts wondering if it was all worth it. I don't want to feel sorry for myself; instead, I'd rather feel that I can find a purpose in life. I understand that this is a big deal and need to search for a solution and find something to keep me occupied and this helps. The idea I have is that I don't just give up, but instead, see what my positive action achieves. Therefore, I am looking for opportunities to take and this is fun.

Looking at what there is on offer and what to avoid is educational. I see how I may need to use my time and skills and create something. It's easier to go out to work for a company or enterprise which is already established but an entirely different thing to establish something from nothing. I am using all my creative imagination to achieve this, among other things, and I don't mind if this is just a way to improve my health. So, I am working on my health to start with because it is not going the way it should. I mean, MS is a very complicated lifelong condition and takes time to manage. Having MS is right in my face and so hard to ignore. I guess rather than ignoring MS and hoping it goes away, I am aiming to put a routine in place to hopefully deal with it in the best way I can. I am not doing this instead of finding a paid job but it leaves me with time to create my own or find a suitable one. Basically, I see my situation as a new beginning and an opportunity to do something new.

The main aspect of this is that unfortunately, things do develop and situations change meaning that my existence was affected by MS. Until my health began to suffer, I thought nothing negative would happen to me. I was completely clueless about how you get MS and although I knew of it by its name, and even knew people who suffered from its effects, I had never asked anyone how you got it and had no real information or knowledge regarding it. Why did I have any reason to have an interest in MS anyway? I really had no idea if it was something you caught or were born with, and I had never thought about that aspect at all. It didn't affect me in my sheltered lifestyle, so why would I need to understand about things that affect other people?

Now, however, because I have since developed MS, I am keen to learn more about it. There are lots of people with MS but I was not going to have the same experience as anyone else – most cases are different. I understand now how it starts, but we don't yet know why or to whom, only that more women than men have it.

MS is typically diagnosed between the age of 20 and 50 and who knows why? I had no idea if I had done something to bring it on or that, in my case, it was the most common type called relapsing-remitting which meant it would come and go. There is plenty of evidence of what happens but not much to explain why. The truth is that nothing can be done for that person until the diagnosis confirms the condition and the process is very in-depth and takes a lot of testing and analysis causing a delay in treatment. In the beginning, the questions I had were all 'why' questions and, as I learned more, I discovered that there are different types of MS and medication, but we still can't answer the question of why we get it.

MS seems to be caused by a malfunction in the immune system but there is no understood reason why this malfunction happens. I hate to say It but I never thought this would happen to me. I did not want it to happen to anyone else; I just did not think it would be me because I was active and well and, therefore, thought the likelihood of anything bad happening to me was so small. So, I guess, being diagnosed with MS came as a shock.

Well, this was a condition I would have to learn to live with so I wasn't going to do nothing. When I learned that I had MS, I started to make changes in my life, and these have continued to this day. Even if health has nothing to do with the condition, it didn't mean that I was going to let my health go to pot. This was not the end – eventually, it could be a new beginning. The main point I need to understand is that I need to do things now and keep active.

Everything changed for me when I was diagnosed with MS for certain and thankfully, I have used the time available to the best of my ability by fully thinking about having MS. The changes I allowed to take place gave me the chance to try and improve my situation. I can't say for sure that I have made the right choices, only that where I am now is a good place considering my old trajectory in life and how I can slowly change it. Basically, I did not like where I was heading and needed to change direction. I didn't want to crash health-wise so needed to make moves and sustain them.

An early diagnosis of any serious condition is essential so don't put your health on hold for any reason - get to a medical professional for a check-up when you feel the need arises. The longer a person puts this off, the more severe the condition may become and therefore the harder to treat. Do yourself a favour and have any lasting symptoms checked out as quickly as you can. I know that people may have responsibilities but I hope everyone understands the need to have a health scare investigated and will allow for a chance to change their commitments to accommodate looking after their health. For example, MS is more common than I thought and most people don't realise this. Hindsight is a wonderful thing so do yourself a favour and get checked out quickly. It took me years to be diagnosed. Time is not always your friend.

It took literally years for my diagnosis, partly because I was unsure of the reason for my symptoms, and just ignored these problems and carried on living with them, so it is possible that I had MS for maybe 5 - 10 years before the diagnosis process even started. I was guilty of thinking my problems would just clear up and never in my wildest dreams thought I had MS. You have to make the first move yourself because how else would the issue be raised otherwise? There are no random MS check-ups that I am aware of, and the process takes time and money, or it did. Really, unless there is first, a reason to suspect MS, and second, an appointment with a doctor about it, I doubt it is ever picked up fast enough. Don't be afraid or feel you are wasting people's time - talk about any issues you have with many people so then a clearer understanding of your health can be reached. If it all turns out to be a false alarm, that doesn't matter. There may be something happening to you that you don't understand, and somebody else may have experienced it with a friend or relative. This can help you emotionally and you will need that help.

Whether your issues are mental or physical, don't keep them to yourself. Find someone to talk to because you don't want or have to go through anything alone. Talking to someone can really help with worry and anxiety too. Whether it's a friend or family member or a professional, or even a cab driver, there are always people to talk to and, eventually, you will gain some useful help. It may be nothing but it's always best to be sure either way. Make sure you find help to deal with whatever is wrong and this will benefit the necessary process.

There were times at school when people commented on my trembling hands but nobody suggested I saw a doctor about it, so I did nothing, and this was a missed opportunity. I should have seen a doctor and pushed for some testing, but I didn't. I did go and see doctors on and off for many years with differing results. When I was younger, the MS was misdiagnosed as a bit of stress so I ignored it when I should have kept going back. Sure, there were missed opportunities, but I have put them behind me and am focused on moving forward with a goal.

It is important to keep mindful of your health which, in my case, was progressively and slowly deteriorating in various ways. The problems I was experiencing were caused because slowly, my immune system was attacking my nervous system and damaging it. Listen, it was very slow and the damage to my nervous system is, to my knowledge, irreversible, but it took time to really become noticeable and on a regular basis. I had no idea what was going on or how it was going to affect me in the long term.

I think a good education must include focus on one's health and well-being to help a person lead a healthy life and be aware if something isn't right; however, when I went to school, this wasn't on the curriculum. I know I must go to the doctor or hospital if there is a major shift in my eyesight or motor functions now, for example. I think most of us would do something too if we stopped walking normally or went blind. The question is, would a person do something if the problems were very slight and slow to appear? With any change, it's important to have the necessary treatment as soon as possible. Now, I wake up every day thinking about my condition and how it is doing, and how I am feeling, and this is needed to ensure I pick up any new problems fast. There is a chance I might go blind in one eye or lose movement in part of my body; it needs to be treated, quickly, with steroids or something suitable to stop the change from becoming permanent. When I go to bed at night, I check myself too. This is probably the last thing I would have done pre-diagnosis because I was young and didn't always even remember going to bed due to my lifestyle. What is wrong with everyone monitoring their health regularly?

The first noticeable symptoms I was suffering were slight and complex, so I thought nothing of them, and years passed before they became an issue in my daily life. With my day-to-day issues being hardly noticeable, and no major change being detected, I did not push doctors to be referred to neurology as I may have if the problems had been major. Given that I had no medical training, I just thought everything was a part of life and my good-for-nothing acquaintances were more interested in ridiculing me about my problems. Even when I was diagnosed, and people knew the diagnosis, there were still some people who showed a lack of empathy, and I am glad I no longer have contact with them.

I also found that I was making bad choices in my life which could have been the cause of some problems with my health, like hangovers due to enjoying clubbing and pubbing a lot, which doesn't help if overdone, and the small symptoms were developing so slowly that I was making likewise adjustments without thinking too much about it, probably because I was living a life of alcohol and late nights and blaming most of it on hangovers. Days went by and I felt normal because any changes were subtle, as were the changes in the way I felt emotionally which were also masked by my lifestyle. I had no major problems and although I went to see doctors with many minor problems over time because none were directly linked to MS, it was never checked. Some things *were* due to MS, and some weren't, but either way, I was undiagnosed and so received no guidance or medication. Nobody knew I had MS for years and years but there were signs there. On more than one occasion, my parents commented on my shakiness but convinced me that it would pass. They could have sought out some advice but did not understand what was going on.

It was nobody's fault, except for maybe a system that lacked the skills and the equipment readily available at that time. The people I knew were no experts in how the body works and I can't blame them for that really. How things change. I needed doctors and neurologists to all come together and assess me but there needs to be a pretty good reason to do this because this is not a standard thing to happen. A proper diagnosis needs time and must consider so many options and possibilities. This is the nature of how my MS behaved and illnesses with similar symptoms need to be considered and ruled out. Back then, even private medical professionals would have needed time to diagnose it. Things have moved on since then and this brings hope for many. At least MS is taken into consideration now when certain symptoms are present where it once wasn't. If you go far enough into history, then MS was not at the same level of diagnosis as in the present time, so by comparison, it is so much better now.

The nerves are used by the body to transport signals to and from the brain to different parts of the body and are a lot like how the wiring in a house transfers energy to appliances. The signals go to and from the brain constantly, even while you sleep, and are important to be there. If I want to move my leg, I think it, and then a signal is sent through the nerves to cause the leg to move. That would be a signal between the brain and muscles to move a body part. If there is damage to the nerve between them, then the signal that is sent between the brain and leg is going to get corrupted by the damage and, in turn, this can cause the task to be affected. Think how faulty house wiring will cause an appliance to not respond correctly. These signals that are being corrupted by damage to the nerve are an indication that there is a problem developing. However, it can be triggered to appear only when a person is tired or hot, which complicates things. I basically only felt the symptoms at times of distress and was otherwise fine. The problems are the things that are picked up and monitored by medical professionals once they are aware of the condition in a case. Identifying that there is a problem in the first place seemed to be the hold-up for me and the sooner the illness was diagnosed, the better because the correct medication could then be used to treat it.

Initially, I didn't think I had any problems, and even when I was diagnosed, I just thought nothing of it. I was living a normal life in my mind and just had a few odd traits. However, the problems were gradually getting worse. Using tests and scans, it is vital to keep records of activity and assess how the body can be treated and these scans weren't readily available back then at the start of diagnosis. I decided that a good way to treat the condition would be with exercise because I thought it would improve my body's health and luckily, I was into exercise anyway. I intend to liaise with my medical team and gain insight into the areas that I think need to be exercised most nowadays and hope they are improved by this. Therefore, I am part of the diagnosis and treatment in so far as I use my test results to work out which specific exercises to use for the various issues.

Of course, I am more aware of my body and how I feel than anyone because I am dealing with it twenty-four hours a day and seven days a week. Due to being at the appointments and being tested physically, I have an idea of what is done and can put myself through similar checks like hand-eye coordination or strength while moving around. I am not trying to replace my medical team who use sophisticated equipment, but instead, work with them in keeping a check on my condition with more awareness. I can offer a daily assessment of my condition and that is more frequent than anyone else. I can keep my own account and tell the medical experts about it at appointments so that they can add the details to my records. My objective is to be as aware of my condition as possible and notice if I have problems that persist. We can then use this information to raise the alarm with the team as soon as possible rather than waiting until my next appointment.

This is a case of cause and effect, where the effects are the symptoms and the cause is the actual illness – that's where the medical professionals come in to try to work this out. The main problem with MS is that there is no cure and so the best thing that can be done is to suppress it as much as possible. I trust that if I do what is needed, then we will have the required information from tests available to treat me for both the effects and the cause of them. After all, MS has changed me and left me with problems that may get worse if the treatment is not sufficient, so I want to be fully treated and not just for the symptoms. For MS, accurately pinpointing the cause and making a diagnosis, then finding the right treatment, can involve a lot of time.

I seem to have been left with an amount of damage to parts of my nervous system which is causing the problems I am trying to cope with; it's all down to the severity of the case for me. Now that I have been diagnosed and am being treated, I am doing well enough and hopefully, if it does get worse, it is a slow deterioration. The more active the problems and the causes are, the more obvious they become, so most of those cases are going to be picked up easier and faster. However, this also means the person is going to suffer more as the symptoms worsen. Every case seems to be different and I think MS is so varied in its behaviour that this is why it is sometimes difficult to diagnose. The sooner MS is picked up, the better the outcome because the sooner it is treated. It can be picked up sooner if the symptoms are more severe, so, it is important to keep going and attend all the appointments and tests you get because, with MS, the problems will keep growing until a good medication is used. I am always looking for the next appointment and expect they will never stop but instead, my illness may become more manageable the more documented it is with the health service. I would be worried if I stopped getting appointments though and would need to do something to make sure I have not been lost in the system as MS is a lifelong condition and needs constant checking.

Only when the diagnosis is made can treatment start, and this is important because the treatment is to slow down the activity of MS so the sooner the better, but it was going to affect my immune system.

Being on a medication that suppresses my immune system is not to be taken lightly because it makes a person more susceptible to infections. Also, the medication used for this itself will cause me some level of discomfort and it may never pass. This was back around the year 2000 when I was around 25, however, it took about five years to become an official diagnosis. Once it was official, I was getting lots of attention from work and friends and made sure I went to all my appointments and cooperated with everybody so was as nice as I can be. As a new case of MS, there was lots of interest in how the condition was behaving because there is so much to learn from each case. I am sure that the whole process is improving and helping people who suffer from MS, and I see it is always moving forward. Basically, my idea is to keep myself going with a healthy lifestyle and exercise alongside everything else the medical experts do because that makes sense rather than leaving it all down to just one arrangement. I am happy to say I have played my part and left the diagnosis and treatment to the medical professionals because that is their part. You see, I want to work on the problem alongside everyone else in whatever way I can, and exercise is a good start. I didn't see it as an option for me to step aside and take a back seat while the experts are involved, but rather, it made me feel less alone and more supported in what I was adding to the program. I can have a lot of appointments to keep up to date with the activity of my MS and the treatment and I am glad for it, and it helps me emotionally to think of all the work taking place.

The MS was starting to affect my walking by this point in time and my balance was being monitored and regularly assessed. The main problems I get are with the temperature and so I suffer most in summer. During the summer, I get up early to exercise while it's still cool. I don't stop exercising because of the temperature and so have just adapted my routine instead. Many years ago, one part of the way to diagnose MS was to put the person in a bath of hot water and see how it affected them, so given that I love and partake in hot baths, I have an idea of how it leaves me feeling. Therefore, I know how the heat affects me, and sometimes I need help to walk so I use a stick or even a friend's arm to hold. I need to think about what I am doing and always check the weather and the distance I will be walking if I go out. Sometimes even crossing the road is too much if I overheat, and I do sometimes get it wrong.

MS is a lifelong condition and will need monitoring and watching and so I am eager to allow this to become part of my life because I want to benefit from this arrangement. I am not going to have any issues with the process that is involved because I understand it must take place to ensure any activity is picked up and monitored, and therefore, I get used to injections and waiting rooms and apparatus which are all involved. I have regular MRI scans too, and these results are compared to previous scan results to look for changes in my central nervous system that are caused by further damage. Damage to my brain will cause problems with my various functions because different parts of the brain control different parts of the body like eyesight or movement. Early detection of further deterioration is important as it gets the professional medical team thinking about treatment and ways to minimize further damage. Everything is regularly checked and monitored for me to get the best outcome as quickly as possible. I spend time going to hospitals to undergo tests and scans and this is so important and must be done. The need for regular assessments keeps my case uppermost and I don't want to be forgotten so I always turn up for appointments. There is also time for me to talk to the medical professionals and that gives me a chance to understand what I am going through and what I can expect and if I can help in any way. The only advice I can get is speculative since we are all different, but that is better than nothing because if there are ways that help me cope, I am all ears. Due to the uniqueness of my MS, I am mainly interested in whether my symptoms will deteriorate or improve, which is hard to say since every case is different. However, no matter the issue, I am always interested in how I can work on my health. I will undoubtedly work on things that are bad and try my best to turn them around. The important thing is to be regularly diagnosed for any changes with MS and understand that any related conditions caused by it may be the result of the medication I am on so take this into consideration too. The whole picture may seem bleak, but I don't let it get to me and use it to create a personalized daily routine that I will use most days to keep me positive. Everything I do needs one hundred percent dedication and so it is important I am keeping positive.

There are new and improved techniques constantly being worked on and it is hopeful that they might benefit me and that future cases will benefit from this as well. I guess that what I am doing in my life sounds like a lot, but I find that come lunchtime, I have moved on and am doing unrelated activities as well. Most things are getting faster and more efficient in the industry now and timely diagnosis is important to help fight this horrible condition so now it is possible that the condition is picked up and treated before it leaves a person in a bad physical way resulting from nerve damage. When I think about it, I imagine what the process would have been like years earlier and the comparison between these two processes. This is a clear sign that progress is being made and this is still helpful for me because the new medication is getting more effective and more readily available. I can only imagine the treatment in the future and how much people will benefit from improved medication and speed of diagnosis. There may come a time when a cure for diseases like MS is found. I experience the effects of MS and they are many and vary a lot, so it is important not to ignore them and instead work on them to overcome them or at least try.

We need to deal with the cause of MS and its effects. First things first, MS needs to be maintained and that means an accurate understanding of the condition must be made and not a generalization. Therefore, after diagnosis, it is key to be regularly checked for changes in the condition, not just for you but also to enlarge everybody's understanding through communication. This is the first stage in getting the best treatment to suit an individual. I am never going to allow myself to get comfortable and so will take every chance to be involved and to help deal with this condition. I want to keep on my toes and am ready to take the necessary action even when it is unexpected or unwanted. Some days, it is a battle to get through and everything seems to be too much. If I don't stay on top of all the appointments I am given, I may miss out on a check-up that turns out to coincide with a deterioration in my health that can be stopped. Nerve damage caused by MS can not be repaired so I need the best medication for me to avoid the damage occurring in the first place, and so far, that is the best option for everyone.

The best way for me to move forward is to cooperate with the medical services and make myself available for whatever is happening. Being diagnosed is only the start of a new task that I must live with and a change in everything I focus on. If I miss an appointment, it may be ages before I get a new one and that is no good. The medical services can be stretched and hard pushed at times and find it hard to make alternative appointments for me, so if, for some unforeseen reason, I miss an appointment, it may be a long time before a new appointment time is available. The best course of action is to reschedule everything else around my appointments and give them priority. If I have anything that clashes with a hospital appointment, then I will reschedule it instead and keep the hospital appointment. It is of utmost importance to stay connected with the arrangement in place between me and the medical team because I want my treatment to be ongoing. I'd rather be unavailable for the repairs to my flat or an annual gas check than a health appointment for I can reschedule them easier so they can wait. As part of my lifestyle arrangements, I am prioritising my health above every earthly thing. If I don't get this right, then I am not going to know how I should react when something changes with my health or medication, and I don't want to take the risk. Being diagnosed with anything as quickly as possible will make treatment and recovery easier and so try to do this all you can. I have put this into place so that I can do just that without thinking. Unfortunately, there may be something that comes up that can't be rescheduled, and in that case, I would choose to miss it which I am very sorry to say. Furthermore, I am always apologetic if I am late and given the worst-case scenario, I will always phone and explain.

There have been lots of twists and turns in my diagnosis, and I can't say it is all easy, but nothing is impossible so stick with it. Since 2000, there have been many people involved in my case and the things I have been through are all part of my MS story. The way my life has been changed and affected by MS physically and mentally is not new. This condition has affected people in the same way for years but the way we treat it is so different and still changing. I have tremendous respect for everyone involved who has given me an opportunity to get where I now find myself - it is not always easy to see where things are going because I don't see into the future. The important thing is that I am here to tell the tale in as much detail as I can recall.

Since my diagnosis was slow, I find it hard to think about all the circumstances at once. I mean, if it had all happened in a few weeks, I would feel upset and overwhelmed but the way it worked out for me, I was able to slowly digest it, take one step at a time and see where things went. I kept positive and still do, which is so important to me now, and this is because it was all new to me making it more of a path down which I had to travel. Nowadays, it comes down to maintaining my connections and being available for tests and check-ups on the medical side which can be a bit less imposing on my life. After all, if you do something repeatedly, it can become routine. I know this is being done for me as my way of life matters. Records are maintained and everything is stable for now; my life has changed, and I now have a health part involving a never-ending commitment from me that I never saw coming. It is wishful thinking that it will end, and I can't imagine a life without all the tests and scans anymore because it has been going on for so long. Still, the Bible does promise, in Revelation 21:4 - "he will wipe every tear from their eyes, there will be no more death or mourning or crying or pain, for the old order of things has passed away." This gives me comfort that a new improved life will come.

I remain impressed by the continued support I am getting from the professionals who are looking after my health needs. It shows they have a real concern for my health and that is why they do the job. I want to see the joy they get from a person coping well and trying hard to do this for themselves too and that gives me motivation. After the first stages of diagnosis, and what felt like going from pillar to post and around the houses, I now feel cared for as far as possible and that any new development in my condition will be picked up and treated efficiently. This has all come from my experiences and has left me with a greater understanding of what is happening and what is being done. Everything I am going through is more than just the experience. What I understand is that the more stable my health is regarding MS, then the less frequently I am required to have an analysis on my condition because my records and evidence of MS support this.

So, there is light at the end of the tunnel. I now feel more confident that my health is not going to deteriorate fast and that I am in good hands. There is a lot involved in the diagnosis of MS and one shouldn't be too worried because it does settle down and become a normal routine with care and diligence. Don't hold back or have doubts no matter how long it takes or what is involved. Just go with the flow and make sure any negative thinking is replaced by a positive attitude. To avoid being forgotten, make your presence felt, keep as many appointments as you can and you will then be given the time to talk over any problems arising from your condition.

I trust the medical professionals and understand they may be under a lot of pressure to meet targets and so I am thankful and show this as best I can. Not wanting to add to their problems, I do everything in my power to help by cooperating. Trust is important and I find it essential to build a good relationship with my medical team and talk with them as human beings. Sometimes I don't understand and get confused and so need to clarify as much as possible, even if I am repeating myself in many ways, however, it is essential to gain clarity. I would be at a disadvantage if I was not learning and using the information I am given.

Being positive is an important part of any treatment and you can help this by staying busy and focused. This world is imperfect, and lots can change and go wrong, so be on the lookout for any irregularities. For example, something might go wrong with the records on the health service side, so it can be helpful to maintain your own just in case. Before I was diagnosed, it was a time of calamity and working overtime at work because I thought money was so important, but now, I have a new strategy and have made changes to enable me to live a rewarding life that is much more enjoyable even though I have a health problem. You see, I would have a health problem any way you look at it. This new strategy has become my focus in life, so if I lose my job, it is okay by me because I now see newly available opportunities where before, it always looked like a persistent problem. Since my diagnosis, my treatment and monitoring have been well-organised so that I can spend time looking beyond the illness and see the new direction in life.

It has taken me much time and there were lots of hoops to jump through but now, three or four appointments a year take care of monitoring my condition. All my health needs are being looked after and I am satisfied with this and will now take other opportunities if I can. This current arrangement may get better or stay the same, and hopefully, if I am doing everything right, I will not get worse. It took a while after diagnosis for things to settle down as it involved a lot of participation, but this now is all part of the process towards a maintainable condition and something I can cope with easily. Although it was not an easy path, I kept going until things settled to being near normal again. I can handle this new arrangement and can spend the rest of my time working on whatever path my life takes me from now on in and moving forward. I have not decided that all that I can achieve is finished; it is more a case of something new that has started to take shape and will keep changing. If this is as far as it can go for now in this direction, if needed, I can take more time to explore other routes and directions. There are lots of directions to take in life and some are still waiting to be discovered. I am comforted to see what the future will bring and know that I can do something with it and not be too restricted. More than anything, I think of overcoming MS and it has almost become a mantra. Let us consider the improvements being made with medication and in diagnosis and how effective and less invasive it all can become, and this can only add to my abilities. These improvements are happening all the time and they are going to become available bit by bit. All that is needed is patience in some respect and imagination in others. So, here is how it was and how it is. The way forward is to always think that I don't need help and although I may get into situations of regret, I struggle, and I keep going. Sometimes I think that I am getting somewhere new which is exciting.

Breaking down the path of my life so far, it falls into three main stages and a fourth emerging. First, there was a pre-MS stage where I lived as a person whose only interests were to enjoy life and live each day as it came, in a pointless, self-satisfying way, leading to a dead end in my opinion. For decades, I was okay and had no health worries. This was okay but at some point, I was going to start having regrets and not seeing anything more to a life of futile existence.

Then came a time when everything gradually went through a major change. It slowly changed due to the development of MS. However, as we have seen, it took many years before a decision needed to be made by me regarding my entire future. Over these years, there was a lot of involvement with medical services and problems with my health being picked up in different parts of my body. The slow onset of the illness gave me time to adjust and understand the gravity of my situation. There came a time of change when I lost a job and couldn't find another and so I had to work on myself for a while.

It is easy to think that my life is over if I am not active, so instead, I stay active to remain sane. It has become necessary to keep my body and mind active throughout every day or get depressed. The work I put in place was to deal with my health and well-being. This takes time and patience but fits in with my medical treatment. I think that I am settled into a routine of exercise and medical treatment and have time to spend on any projects I like. I am mainly busy every day with the routine I have established and anything that happens to benefit my health is down to the advancements in medicine and my fitness. Thankfully, my condition is stable except for the occasional ups and downs that may be caused by a virus or the like. Sometimes, things seem to be going in many directions at the same time and I can only spend time in meditation and prayer about how everything will turn out. I mean, whether a medical improvement is achieved to repair the damage, or my exercising and diet give me back what I have lost, or of course, it could be a combination of everything I am doing for myself, whatever happens next, I want to be around to see it.

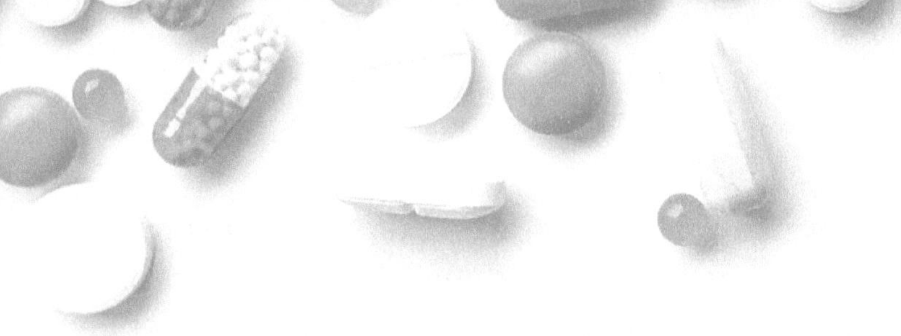

CHAPTER 2

With the help of medicine

MS is where the immune system is misbehaving and it is attacking the nervous system. Therefore, most medications for treating MS these days suppress the activity of the immune system, which is the cause, and unfortunately, this can also increase the risk of catching viruses such as the flu or Covid for example, and so has its issues. To be honest, most medications have issues with dosage and the associated amount of side effects. So, it is understandable to realise that all medications do have their drawbacks and with mine, the heightened risk of infection is one, so it is beneficial to get the flu vaccine and Covid vaccine than suffer the damage caused in the long term if I take nothing. Anyway, these vaccinations for flu and Covid are a good thing to stop people from being ill, especially the elderly and very young.

Immune suppressants are readily available now for treating MS, depending on the severity of the case, and are effective for me, so I take the type of suppressant that is the most suited to me and I live with its side effects. I am not an expert on my medication for MS but what I have is trust in my medical team to work this out based on my tests and their expertise. I don't feel that I am overcoming MS thanks to the medication that I take but it only improves my condition if I take it and do what I can to help too. Therefore, I am pleased that I am mostly okay.

I understand that there are different immune-suppressing drugs available and that not everyone's MS responds to the same medication in the same way. What I won't do is stop taking my medication and this is important even though the side effects may make me feel bad. If I take medication for long enough, I generally get used to its side effects and I know it is important that people give their treatment a chance before giving up on it. I am sure that my current medication is doing more good than harm so I leave myself strictly under the guidance of professionals.

There are always new variations being developed and I need to weigh up the pros and cons of changing. Of course, I can always stay on what I am taking and that is down to me having the final say, however, I want to keep up with newer and better medication and so usually change. I ask about the new medications to find out the efficacies and methods of how they are taken to help me decide. After all, I don't want to end up taking the wrong medication because it is too involved a process and I can base this on previous experience I have had with medications that require a lot of involvement. There is more to it than just taking the strongest available as this can involve invasive procedures that are too inconvenient. My aim is to find the most effective medication with the least side effects. Obviously, I can't have everything and so consider the medication closest to my liking.

Medication must build up in effectiveness and it is important to get this right when changing medication. Do not start with the last resort and most powerful medication because the medication needs to be tailored to your case. The best way to find the most suitable is by beginning at the bottom and increasing the dosage until it is right for your condition. If you start at the top level unnecessarily, that will leave you with nowhere to go, so unless this is the only option, leave the choice to the professionals because it is a difficult one. This is why I leave the choices up to my medical team as they are the ones with the knowledge and experience.

Take the medication you need to deal with your health problems, but also, give it time to work because the medication doesn't cure MS instantly but works on reducing its activity. As and when it is advised or appropriate, try something more powerful and give it a chance to work to the best of its ability. Don't just give it a day and then change it for something else because of how it makes you feel. I was patient and tried what was available for my treatment, a drug which had the least impact on how I felt and was something I could work with as directed by the medical team. So, in the beginning, I was just started on muscle relaxants to steady the spasms in my eyes because that was all that was needed. I also gave that medication time to work and only changed my treatment when I could benefit in some way that was more to deal with MS since the muscle relaxants were dealing with just the symptoms. Again, unless there is a good reason to change the medication, like it is causing bad reactions, I try to stick to my treatment for two years. There needs to be a pretty good reason to change my treatment without giving it a good chance to work. Soon I found a treatment that suited me because it treated the cause of MS, and I was left on the medication for the reduction of nerve damage. I need both medications for the cause and effects of MS and so need to manage a lot of tablets each day. There is a possibility that the treatment may be made more effective through medical advances and this may be something to discuss with your medical team. I am interested in new breakthroughs for treating multiple sclerosis and talk to my neurologist about these during appointments. I involve myself in all my treatments and try to understand how they work. The medication may work and leave you with no new activity but you must keep taking it or the activity will restart. Then there will always be the problems you get from nerve damage like spasms and loss of functions which need treating and that medication is going to have to continue.

All medication, I have found, comes with side effects whether I feel them or not and so they seem to all need regular blood tests to identify them. There are some medications that I have taken which have given me hot flushes too and to various degrees. As we have already discussed, I don't like feeling hot because it disables me, so if I get hot, I need to get somewhere to cool off. When hot, I lose coordination and strength in various parts of my body so a flush or fever is most unwelcome. The heat inflames my nerves which further interferes with signals. I love hot baths though and need to take necessary precautions when I take one and so I always hydrate before, during and after and then I empty the bath before I get out and try to cool down a bit. I have had a grab rail fitted to support me when in the bath and shower which is a must. I am prepared to endure almost any heat and compensate by drinking fluid during the day, and after a hot bath, I always allow a few days to fully recover.

Then there are the silent side effects where they are stealthily creating havoc with my internal workings like brain and heart function. These side effects need to be checked by a professional. I seem to need to take blood tests and blood pressure and pulse checks a lot. The results are recorded and enable the health professionals to check that there are no problems caused by the medication I am on that could be dangerous. All in all, I always seem to get a combination of side effects, and therefore, I take care of myself with a routine that fits in with the medical professional's checks. It seems to depend on the individual how the side effects of a medication may cause them distress but there are mitigating measures we can all take. I try to put up with side effects and get used to them and wait till something better becomes available by keeping fit and healthy in a way that also helps me to cope with my feelings. There may be days where it is worse than others and it is not wrong to maybe take paracetamol to take the edge off the discomfort. This is sometimes the only option but I try not to do it too much. Interestingly, exercise seems to break the headaches I get.

To control MS, I started on a medication that needed to be injected into my flesh three times a week and it had side effects that gave me a raised temperature like the flu does sometimes (lucky me). Having checked that it was okay to do so, I experimented with taking the medication at different times of the day. Taking it at the end of the day so I slept through most side effects was an option I tried for a while and changing times to see how I coped best gave me something to do. The medication needed to be kept in my fridge to keep it useable because a higher temperature would mean it could lose its effect. It was not possible to take it orally either because the stomach acids would destroy it. Again, it was an injection, and I was trained by a nurse and then was on it for several years. I didn't like the lumps or bruising that appeared caused by regular injections and occasionally, I would cause a small bleed, but that goes with the fact of injecting so much. As advised, I varied the sites that I injected into to reduce damage to my flesh and that worked. I started on a syringe with a small amount of fluid for my body to get used to it and then increased to the full dose after two weeks. This meant more fluid to inject but not more often thankfully. It came with a device you could load up and it would fire the syringe and inject me to make life easier, however, if that device broke, I needed to do it by hand so was trained to just in case. After years of taking this medication, I found that I would just inject it by hand anyway for the speed because I was so used to the injection procedure.

The medication needed to be kept at a low temperature so if I wanted to travel, then I kept it in a bag with ice packs and lots of stuff like travel bags all came with the medication. I include taking my medication in my normal routine, just like brushing my teeth; it is just something I need to do so I just get on with it. Taking medication regularly may come with its own obstacles, however, no matter the struggle, I get used to it over time. You may hear of alternative treatments that you can look at, such as healings, etc., however, I know full well that Satan is the father of lies and wants us to follow him to ruin. I will not make a big mistake and stop medicating without an alternative and better treatment that has been proven and is available at that time from my medical team. Therefore, I am involved with my health professionals for advice on such matters and don't take it upon myself.

Disease-modifying therapy is the name of a treatment that suppresses the immune system and stops it from overreacting. When I started on disease-modifying therapy, I needed to administer it myself by way of injections because that was the only available action at that time, so, I just got on with it and I took it for several years and got used to it. There were a few types of medication to choose between and they all needed injecting at that time and in different ways. I watched a video on each type of disease-modifying therapy, and some looked very frightening to take in the way they were injected, and then I settled on one which I felt most comfortable with. I held on though it was an effort and the treatment available changed, so it did pay off eventually to be patient and endure situations, and not give up. After all, it took a few years before my medication was available in tablet form. A wait without treatment may have caused the condition to worsen. As soon as tablets became available, I took the opportunity to switch and was much happier with that move because it turned out the tablets also had the bonus of better efficacy, and the side effects had less of an impact even though there were some. However, nowadays, I am used to most of them.

We are all different and new therapy may cause changes for some. I remember this change mostly because it made a big difference in my quality of sleep which improved a lot. When I take medication less regularly, there is more of an up and down to its effect, so the more regular way fits me because the effects are smoother. I still got the effects of flushing though which is only a problem when I am sleeping. On occasions, I would wake up drenched in sweat which got me out of bed, and I needed to be cooled off. That is an improvement for me, and it is just a matter of taking the tablets and not forgetting. I was normally okay because a hot flush during the day just turned me red. Eventually, those side effects became something I didn't really notice.

There are so many medications available for MS, and it will take time to find the best for me which will involve trying different ones. Given the time I have been on MS medication, I am sure that I am benefiting from it even if it is not the most suitable yet. I am thankful that currently, there are options that are good, and I am sure that new and improved medications are being developed that may be closer to the mark. The medication is my hope for treating MS and having it under control, so I make sure I take it and get used to the idea. MS is a serious problem and will never go away, therefore, I will need to stay on medication unless it becomes possible to stop MS from being active and repair the damaged nerves it has left me with. Even if the medication I take stops any MS activity, I will still need medication to stay on top of the illness and help me feel better. I can't see into the future and so I can't see how my condition will go but I can see into the past and how medication has progressed over my life. The hope that medication is constantly improving is good news for many and I will not dismiss it as impossible. I do know that I am now required to take medication and need to live with that fact. I think that there comes a time when the condition of MS stops and that the next stage will be reversing the damage caused by it. From the condition to the health problems it leaves me with, there is medication to help me feel better. Look, I didn't see this happening, but the scans show it, and I am trying to be optimistic every day of my life. The truth is, I don't want to spend too much time thinking that I will be cured because I have a job to do and medication helps; a job to live and keep living and that takes lots of work. I must take medication and do my best to deal with anything that this illness throws at me not forgetting the basics. I can use any extra time I have in other ways.

I am aware that the medical industry is working around the clock on the treatment of MS and nerve damage. The work being done by pharmaceutical companies covers all manner of health conditions and MS is just one of them and this is good for humanity. If medication becomes available and is suitable for me, I will be thankful and make the move. The chance of new and improved medication becoming available is improving with time and I try to remain optimistic and patient. The hope this gives me helps me continue with every part of my life and it affects me with purpose and direction. I must remember how far the treatment has come along and use this thought to give me a way to imagine how fast it is improving and can get. The medication I am on now wasn't available when I was first diagnosed and is an example of the improvements being made. If I think about it, I must consider that the work will not stop until a solution is found. I am hopeful that the medication will progress enough to help everyone no matter the state they are in.

Feeling satisfied that medication is working to combat the MS in me and that I can leave it to the professionals while I carry on with life is a blessing. I have been on medication to treat MS long enough to accept it as part of life and I know that I need it to deal with the illness that is MS. I can't imagine a time when there will be a complete recovery for me, and this is no longer something I look forward to but that is because I am realistic and know that it would be a miracle if it happens in my time. I used to think that I would return to normal, and I can't think like that anymore because it has gone on for too long, so I am doing my best just to survive. I guess that is the harsh reality of life and I am glad of my belief and understand there is more to life than what I thought as a secular young person. I am down with the illness and have faith to help me deal with it. God bless.

Just as Covid-19 hit, I was beginning a treatment that was to be taken by infusion in hospital once every six months, so this arrangement proved impractical and I decided to change to a more suitable one. This may have been a chance missed on my part, but in the end, I had to put my foot down and say that the infusions were just not going to be practical because of the pandemic because they had to be preceded by blood tests which were being delayed by Covid issues and so I stopped that medication and arranged a different one.

I only thank our heavenly Father for that prophecy and have no regrets. The efficacy of the new medication that I turned down was much better than the one I was on and it would have been good to stay on it and may have been a game-changer, but such is life, and it gave me more understanding of the choices in medication. Due to Covid-19, the waiting times were increasing drastically, and I was not getting the dose required as a result even though it was the early days of the pandemic, so I had a bad feeling about it. I had to consider the disruption to the treatment and compare it with the medication I was on and luckily, there are always alternative medication options nowadays. Due to this exact problem, I now find it useful to ask how I take the treatment and the details of the regularity, etc. I just didn't see the pandemic in time or think of a way through it without my treatment being disrupted. From this experience, I am interested in a treatment that I can take myself and how I get it, and this is probably due to events that are out of anybody's hands, so I try to think of a best-case scenario. Tablets tick all the boxes for me nowadays and many medications come in tablet form now and so I am leaning toward them. They can be delivered to my door too and I do the rest. Once again, I'm so glad for the advice and support of my medical team who are extremely helpful and understanding when it comes to situations such as these.

I am always thankful to hear about advancements in the treatment of MS being made and I get posts from the MS society which keep me informed. I am satisfied with the therapy I am on because I feel okay about it keeping the advance of MS down and thus giving my body more recovery time. This is because with relapsing-remitting MS, the time it remits for is better the longer it lasts, and this is when MS is not attacking my nerves, so control is welcome. I would rather have some medication that reduces the activity than none. There are always risks and side effects, so I have regular tests and keep an eye on myself daily to see how I am holding up just in case my medication becomes a problem and stops working properly.

One of the most important things with illnesses such as MS is continuity of car – make sure you take your medication regularly and always ensure you have a supply available for holidays, days away, etc.

I am always asking my medical team about the advancements in the repair of damage to the nervous system when a new medication becomes available. If this becomes a reality, it will help so many so much and would be a game-changer for sure. The important thing is that I don't give up my routine and spend time dreaming about cures for the nerves that have been damaged. Not that doing that is wrong but there are more important things that I need to prioritise. Still, repairing damaged nerves is a game-changer for sure and would help many conditions and not just MS and that is why work continues with it. Until such medication is available, it is business as usual, so I leave it with the professionals who work tirelessly on such things while I work on my strength and stamina. I am being realistic and doing my bit to keep my health at a good level.

At the moment, the medication I take is over fifty per cent effective, so the drugs are working, and my life has settled down allowing me to catch my breath, so to speak, and modify my life where necessary. It has been a long time coming and I hope it lasts and gives me a chance to focus on a routine to build strength and stamina which I don't want to neglect. Therefore, my journey was long, and I needed to stay with it to gain some normality and feel emotionally better. I know what I am doing when it comes to taking medication, so I have now got a medical routine and it fits in with my life well.

Some days can be too hot for me, which is funny because I used to love summertime, however, I still try to do what I can. I need to be somewhat prepared and flexible in case my health changes so a level of preparedness is an important part of anything. A person needs to accept things change over time and be okay with this but be prepared for sudden changes too. It has happened to me before, and the important thing is I was willing to adapt even though it happened rather fast at times. The main changes occurred at the beginning of getting diagnosed but if you give it time, you will benefit in the long term. A person can be ready for changes and be capable of dealing with them but it is also vital to look at things you can do to help yourself, such as through positive activity or exercise. It is also important to increase rest to help you cope with changes.

If something needs to be done to maintain my health, I am ready to jump into action with the knowledge and belief that I can handle things. Like a coiled spring, I realise how important it is not to panic when there are changes, and not to get comfortable if there are no changes but to find a middle ground instead. I am ready to act sensibly with care and consideration. For better or worse, I will do the necessary to maintain the status quo in my life and each day I wake up, I first give thanks for another day to work with. I keep positive because there are days when things go wrong but there always have been. This is a long road I'm on with no way to know what is on it, so I am doing my best to stay on the road and keep moving past any obstacles along the way. I guess this sounds a lot like a normal life. I am going the distance, maybe not at speed, and will keep it up because the chance to do this is in my hands and I am willing to do my best.

Sure, I could just think there is nothing I can do but that is not the case because I can exercise. I regularly take medication because I am convinced I need to, and it is a part of my routine, so if the medication changes, I need to become accustomed to the new medication in all it brings and that may take a few years, but I don't need to sit on the bench for that either and I get up and join the proceedings. Sure, the side effects may be a challenge and I won't let that stop me. These changes can bring an improvement in the way I feel and can prove to be a blessing and give relief when the body is used to them. Sometimes, we can find that previous medication no longer brings the benefits it used to because it loses its effectiveness so I have to be prepared to change in this scenario.

Anyway, I am prepared to do what is needed when it comes to my health and the medication is part and parcel when it comes to MS. Any serious illness must be a daunting prospect and you must keep busy living so do your best to keep living in a satisfying way. Be aware that we are all imperfect and that these obstacles are trying us.

Over the years, whenever something new becomes available that might benefit my situation, I have been given the chance to try it. However, I have the final say. I can take time to think and research it all if I want. I know that the medication is being used successfully before I am offered it and that is reassuring. It is important not to be put on a medication that is too powerful or not powerful enough and it is sort of in-between. The process of finding what is best for you may take time and will work out eventually so stay with it and keep pushing for more inclusion with everything, but be aware, these things can take time. It can be a fight to endure some of the trials when speaking about new medication or treatments, but things just happen that way. A person with beliefs must keep going and not stop and wait for a different option to become available - after all, how will we know how long that will take?

As it stands, my MS is stable and there is no deterioration in my health that can be noticed and so it means I just need to stay on the medication under the close supervision of my medical team. There has always been a level of medication suitable for me to help me maintain a normal life. Again, I am thankful that science is there to supply what it can. Although there are lots of opinions and advice that people offer, I will not let myself be coerced in a direction other than that of my medical team. I can add things to my routine, but I will not remove anything because I have gone through some major shifts in life and where I am is sufficient.

I know there are people who choose to do only as they please and there are dangers to this in all walks of life. Although there are lots of alternative options out there, I think the medical route is the one for me after careful consideration. From my research, none of the alternatives stand up on their own. Be careful not to get conned or scammed and always listen to the professionals and get as much advice as possible to develop the most rounded viewpoint. For example, holistic medication would not be my immediate choice but is an option to consider alongside the medication path. I could try to deal with MS without medication, but I choose to include it in a routine of fitness and diet instead. I have prayed about it and researched the action to take medication and am happy with my decision. Obviously, it is down to the individual in the end. It all starts with what makes me happy, and if I am happy taking medication, then I don't need to abstain. The decision to take medication is something I may live with for a long time, and I have thought about this too and come to terms with it. I will continue with this approach and see what happens.

Medication does not mean a risk-free option because there are always risks, for example, if the instructions aren't followed. Consider that there is a danger in every action, like crossing the road for example, and this gives you a full understanding. The thing is, some actions are riskier than others. Try to be well informed before you take any leap and know the risks of doing it and equally not doing it. Whether it's acupuncture or some holistic treatment I have, I would still take my medication as well. I would suggest clean living of the mind and body can help. Meditation and prayer can be a regular addition to daily life as well as a healthy diet and hydration. Now, I like to exercise for about an hour a day and the more I do, the more I can do, so there is a lot more going on than simply taking medication. It is tempting to stop exercising during the summer because of the heat but I push through and when the weather changes, I see the improvement I have made by not stopping. It sounds like a lot of activities, but I have built it up from a simple exercise routine I did three times a week when I had a job and exercising is still a major part of my life. The funny thing is I am using the situation I am in to do the most I can with my time and if I found a job, I would need to change everything I have put in place. However, if that becomes a necessity, I can adapt my routine to fit around a job while still maintaining the healthy living choices I use today.

I have got to take medication even when I am ill and so medication is the first thing I focus on. I don't really know if my body is recovering but I get a sense that it is. Even if my condition stopped completely, I would still seek advice and follow the directions of my medical team. I have stopped telling people how I am doing and instead tell them the medication I am on, and they can decide the rest for themselves. The truth is, the medication I take is a major contributor to my condition and that is all. Without the medication I take, I don't think that I would be as well as I am after all this time. Sure, I could abstain from medication and feel better but for how long? All things considered, the longer I stay on medication the better. I mean, the longer I don't take medication, the worse my health will get and there is no way to repair nerve damage, so it is more about how I function than how I feel. The side effects and everything I experience from taking medication are well worth tolerating to me. When dealing with MS, it is necessary to do everything you can and get used to it. Think of the benefits and not the negatives.

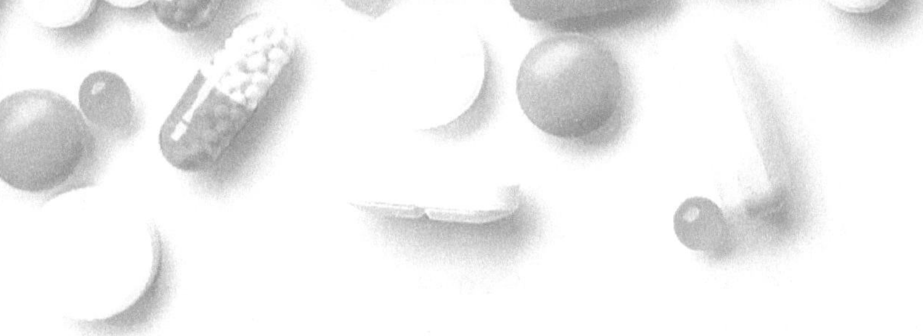

CHAPTER 3

An end to the old ways of life

I couldn't go on with my life as it was anymore because it was like I was my own enemy, and I was born into a system of life dictated to me by the part of the world I live in and those around me. I could only look at how my parents and peers lived their lives and was unaware of any other options available to me. I felt that I was trapped into following the crowd and fitting in with them. I was also unaware of all the chances I could take if I decided not to just conform.

I like to think back and remember all that I can and see how things have changed and what I have been through. I always had the urge to break away but was afraid I would be alone because I was told not to do anything other than what society taught. I think my feelings were too strong at times and I remember arguments with my mother and friends, where it seemed like I was wrong and they were right. I think it probably is just a difference of opinions and a lack of self-control that causes most arguments. My parents always told me how different it was when they were young and how it is now; I get it. When they grew up, there wasn't MTV or mobile phones. I guess you need to live some before you can reminisce, but you get to a point when there is lots to look back on. So, wherever you are, it may be a different society and way of life, but it is what you think of as normal and, in essence, has its own memories. This is great if we gain experience from it, but not all changes are bad so they might be worth considering.

We all have a story to tell. The interesting thing is, historically, a lot has changed and not all to the good. Take the Bible for example, because it contains lots of proven facts and shows us how we have lost paradise in pursuit of wealth and power. This is the big picture, and I am talking about me in it and how I just represent a speck of time that I am from, so please understand this is all I represent in the cosmos. I haven't always done my best or been happy and that may have been caused in part by a view of the system I was in and my feeling that there must be more to life. I am not happy to think that this is as good as it gets. I needed to find a purpose long before I got carried away with the nine-to-five working life malarkey. I remember that I was so much freer when I was young than I became through society, so I question the changes. I want to feel young again and carefree and all because I feel I have lost something precious without it. Unfortunately, it is hard to feel that way all the time. However, doing nothing but existing is not good for anything else and I want to try to turn a trajectory that is hopeless into hopeful, and this is a start. It all can be an adventure and I think I want a change made with a reinvented life.

Things in my life were average at best and my life fitted in with how I was brought up to believe it was supposed to be, so I needed to start fresh. I guess I wanted to fit in with the world and live a life that was ordinary and when I think about it, I see how pointless that attitude is and how it needed to be changed. The thing is, I was comfortable with a life that had become a passing of time and just felt comfortable. Lots of people are happy with comfortable and that is fine until then something like ill health affects it and causes you to rethink everything. Comfortable is sufficient but there is something in me that would not settle for that or return to it. I spent most of my time trying to think of things to do while watching TV or listening to music which is doing nothing and futile. If I'm honest, a big part of my life was turning into a huge waste of time with the occasional weekend away. How futile is it to take the gift of life and just throw it away? I exercised somewhat and ate reasonably well and there was no reason for this behaviour other than to increase the amount of life I could waste. That is the funny thing about it all. Think about it; the days went by like a futile exercise in enjoyment just living for the weekend when I would hit the pubs and clubs to enjoy alcohol and music. Occasionally, I went away for a change of scenery and that was about it because mostly, I was doing as little as possible in the many days in between and these were the days that held the opportunities. The opportunities were what I realise was a chance to really make something out of my life. I spent some time in evening classes and that didn't amount to much other than some qualifications and that is it. I think my MS was what stopped that from continuing more anyway. I can't imagine where I would be if I hadn't developed MS, which is slowly taking over my life and changing the direction it was heading, and I mean that in a somewhat good way. Maybe I would have achieved a higher level of qualifications and gained more responsibility and a better wage still in the rat race, but I prefer the challenges I am facing now which you can only understand through experience.

However, was this where my life was going? I didn't know how long it was going to last with the lifestyle I had been living anyway. Something was not right if this was how I was leading a life pre-diagnosis. I see so much through the internet which will tell you what you want to hear, when you boil it down, about what I was doing with my life and how I was becoming so used to it that I thought it was all okay. This is saying that my life is filled with normality and nothing to worry about so get comfortable. I was heading nowhere fast and yet everything was telling me that this was what I should do and it was okay. Nothing memorable and plenty to tut at was all that could be truthfully said about all that I had achieved. All this time, I was missing out on so much and thought the opposite was true and so I carried on regardless. It is pathetic to think that I had everything I needed and so I should stop looking for the next move and instead just enjoy as much as possible. Thankfully, I didn't leave it too late and can say that I am on the right track now. If I had let society have its way, I would have given up on having dreams and ideas outside of the box. This is where it is important to get the facts and not just opinions. I don't want to give up and just live in a meaningless and unsatisfying way.

As a teenager, I left education and went out to work and it was as simple as that; this is what people did and what I understood I was to do. Maybe I should have followed my desires as early as possible but instead, I worked for employers and myself over the years. I would get up then go to work and then come home only to do the same again the next day. This went on and this is how I would have spent my entire life because I didn't know any better, but I have always felt the desire to be more, and it is a shame I did nothing with it. It may be that I was so wrapped up in enjoying myself that until I grew up a bit, I didn't want to take life seriously. Working for money is a dead-end way for me to spend my life because I always wanted more from my time while I was working. I had no idea there were so many rewarding ways to live. There are so many things I could have spent my time doing. I hate to say I had a level of fear about being out of work and having to fend for myself. There were even a few reckless years where I was working six days a week and fitting into it a social life and that was just leaving me stressed and tired, so I got out by doing what I do best and stopped trying to please my employers. The six days were not all spent in one job so I had to spend time working out what job I was doing and when which was very stressful. The more, I got to know employers, the more I saw how greedy and uncaring they are when you push them to answer that. All my employers over the years started off nice at initial interviews but seem to find fault in me and a reason to treat me with less kindness as time passed as if they only feel for new people and not for those they'd known for longer.

I also don't think you deserve any friends if you lose interest in them as I did; instead, concentrate on building up good friendships. I think the more you know people, the more you are a friend to them, and friends should treat their friends like themselves. I now realise that there is a more enjoyable life I can cultivate that is including something different than just work, rest and social life. I understand that we all have a chance to live a fulfilling life and society only encourages us to get a job and earn money and try to live out our lives and that is it. When I think about this, I realise that this is so we all pay taxes and contribute to society to keep it going. What I chose to do wasn't ever noble or selfless and so that is what I needed to change. I was on board with this work mentality so much so that it was what I had settled into, and it would take a major event to change that. I forgot that I could make choices and I had gotten comfortable with a life of such futility and there was a risk of that becoming everything I wanted to do. It was good to have experience and qualifications, and this showed, so I decided to put my time into a career, and yet, no matter how much I achieved, the inevitable is unavoidable. Sometimes I need to consider these things and that is needed to keep me feeling there is an extra option. We are all different and I wish good luck to everyone who is travelling this mortal coil in their chosen way.

My crime is that I let myself become a piece of furniture. I had forgotten to have a purpose, and I was not pushing anymore and instead, was just coasting along. I had been blinded by everything in the media and led astray with lies and had forgotten the gift life is. The roles I was doing were not changing except when the software I used was updated and that was the only time I needed to really use my head. I would, from time to time, need to learn what had been changed at work and how it impacted my workload and that was it. I didn't know any better and thought what I was doing in doing a job was what everyone did and so left it at that. As far as I was aware, the option was simple, and I went along with it. Sometimes it is important to step outside yourself and view yourself as someone else does and that way see you have options. See that you are wasting time in jobs where there is no fairness. Maybe a realisation will create courage for changes to be made.

In my life, I was caught in a snare because, in retrospect, I know it was not all there is, but I thought that it was and was blind to so much. The only people I was making happy were those who were making money from my work. I am sorry to all those who thought I should have given up instead of persisting in work with a disability and I didn't listen because I needed to consider the alternatives. The thing is, work was all I knew and was a safe option and the only option I could think of until I needed to make a complete change. I had no inkling of all the things I was missing out on and, due to being narrow-minded, I didn't think of being able to do other things instead. I needed to rally, be ready to go, and it took years to feel that I had more reasons to go than stay. Changing my life, a lot seemed like so much effort and I doubted I could do it and I needed to believe in myself. I thought a lot about my past to see what was of use.

As I grew up and went to school, they would ask me what I wanted to do when I grew up and then educated me on what lessons I needed to go on and do well in. Finance is my discipline and what I do; this needed a certain skill, and I never made any real choices myself and just went to my lessons and sat my exams. However, I was getting complacent after years of working and my ill health wasn't helping. If I didn't realise that I had potential then, I do now. It takes a person's strength to decide that they can change their whole situation and the courage to do it and escape to something new. We're not talking about just moving jobs - I needed to revaluate my entire life.

I am more satisfied working and doing my best now that I have changed my old life for a new one. I graduated as a life coach and now know there are fundamental things that must be done, whatever you do, like exercise to maintain physical and mental health. A healthy diet and hydration are needed for life and there were times I got this wrong due to work environments, but now I know better. I needed to consider the worst-case scenario and not be afraid and so I let my job leave me and that is the best way to explain what happened there. On the one hand, I could get comfortable and live out my days doing an ordinary job and that would be that, but I jumped out of that while I was able to make the change. The old life I was in was being changed by health issues and I wanted to put that in a better situation. As it turns out, I was able to use it and create a life that benefited me rather than just supported me. I need to find a way to benefit my health and provide a living. I don't think going to work every day was giving me the best shot at a reasonable life, all things considered. I was losing interest in my life, and it was time to do something about that anyway. I needed to start living again and this was a big deal and involved changing a lot. Facing the future with not much to look forward to is not good but I am doing my best and turning that prospect around. I need to feel alive and purposeful. I want to put my old life behind me and move forward with my new life in a total restart. I may need to make sacrifices and see what opportunities are available and so what if I need to go through some rough patches? Sometimes things go your way if you just let go of the old life you lead and try something new.

When I found myself in a life which was gathering dust, I had become an empty vessel and I felt stuck in this system, but out of the darkness, I found hope. I needed to make a new situation and be strong in making a new start even when sometimes I would feel completely stuck. How did I feel about the state I was in? Well, basically, I was a person with no insight and no ambition. I was a person who had lost all my drive and interest and I had fallen into a set routine and thought I was happy while I had a job. I was just existing and lacked any real purpose, so I needed to do something about it. What made it difficult was that I was alone with nobody to turn to. If I didn't do something new, then my life was going to pass by and away leaving me in a coffin and forgotten. This may happen anyway, but I feel so much better that I am doing something meaningful with my life now. I did not want to just wait for the inevitable to take place. What I was doing for work wasn't very special either -anybody could do it, so I didn't really care when it finished. I don't think they liked me much anyway and I got that impression when I left. There were probably a few who were happy to see me go. They may feel important, but they aren't, and they never will be to me; no great loss. Loads of people are living a life in this way and I can't see the benefits anymore. I would like people to have a revelation and start doing something about it before it is too late. This was my situation, and, in my gut, I wanted to change... like a caged animal wants to escape.

I craved something new, and I knew it wasn't going to be easy, especially now, but I took each day at a time. I was lucky in the fact that I had the time and the inclination to do something else so away I went. I was in a cycle of work that others benefited from, and I would still be today if I hadn't stood up for myself and taken no part in someone else's money-making affairs. It is important to get away from people who don't care much about me and are only interested in possessions because this can rub off on me and I am happy with the basics. Maybe I brought this on myself and maybe I escaped from it because I had gained an awareness of myself before it was too late. I have time and drive in me and can use them instead of putting them aside and just carrying on with the old way. I think it is best to put some things behind me and stop them or fair badly. The transition from a life that I had grown used to is far from easy and needs sacrifice and work, so it took time. I needed to use courage and lots of it because I needed to make major changes and use strength. My situation helped as I was just working on being me and personally involved with nobody else to worry about or depend on, but I still needed to do it a bit at a time because it was going to be too much altogether. So as and when I can, I am working on stopping bad habits which are harmful. I need to ask myself why I do this and lots of questions like that. Also, I ask myself what a better use of my time is.

I spent about thirty years running around in circles and look where it got me! Then I finally got away and now it gets interesting. So what if I have MS to deal with? That is something I need to deal with no matter what I do. Don't fall into the same trap... instead, find a real reason to look after yourself and others with an understanding of who will be there with you when you need help. The world is in a really bad situation, and I will be better on my own for this work. Look, I feel like I have been trapped without any freedom to express myself in retrospect and only now I am free. However, everything I have been through has given me experience and I only now realise it can be of some use and help me move into something new. I have realised that I can use all the long and boring days and the numerous people I have dealt with as a source of knowledge to my advantage and also use having MS too. Everything has had a purpose and even if I didn't realise it at the time, I have gained from all of it. Yes, the good and bad times are all useful. I am fortunate that I got out while I did and didn't waste too much of my life pursuing the pointless dead-end life anymore and that having MS has given me a purpose to survive and use the experience in some way.

So now, I am going through my new reinvented system and getting a benefit from all my life so far, a benefit that I never realised was possible until I gained a new purpose in life. The work that I do has escalated, and I find that I am now busy and enjoying it because it is like a new start and a breath of fresh air. Sure, I have a big obstacle I am constantly trying to surpass but I am finding it a useful experience. The times I've spent with someone looking over my shoulder and commenting on me are gone and not forgotten because I can see the error and a solution. All my life experiences are of use to me, and I am reminiscing lots, and it is wonderful. Sometimes I apply for jobs if there is a suitable position and would do the work if I got the job, so I haven't totally given up. There would need to be some stipulations, however, that I would need to meet, and I need to consider fully what I am getting myself into first. My choice would be more mature than the way I operated historically but that is due to what I was and what I have become. I don't even seem to be getting interviews anyway so now it is just speculation and can wait for a while. There is a lot going wrong in the world like disease and inflation and war. I am happy to work on my own for as long as I need until I am totally ready to do something else.

It is important to understand the difference between n old life and a new one so that I can let go of living the old life and start living the new one with ease. Obviously, there is a time of transition between the two states, and this is really the time when the old ways are becoming the new ways of living. I just can't believe the way I lived my life and am sorry that I didn't do something about it sooner. A new life is full of possibilities and has so much more to offer but I am in no rush to do things that are in danger of going wrong if not done well. You see, I need to work out what I am going to stop and what I am going to start or just adapt. It is important to plan and work on a new life to make sure it is going to be correct and that any errors are small and easily sorted out.

Looking back, I have regrets and think I can learn how not to do certain things again as a result which is useful. Now my new life involves a lot of planning and I think any major changes will need to be worked on so I expect I will need time to adjust. Obviously, some things will take more time than others but it is way more important to get things right than making a few temporary sacrifices because of the time it takes. My skills, though, stay with me and do not get left behind and so I have these tools available. Of course, there will be elements that are similar, and this can help to speed up settling into a new life where there are going to be completely new things to learn as well, and these need more involvement.

Especially if you have lived your old life for a long time, some changes can be harder to make because of the effort involved, so make sure you weigh up the best ones to change. It has taken time with me, and I have worked hard just to move on and leave my old ways. I have also worked hard to get my new ways in place.

Believe me, it takes a lot of thinking and planning to set yourself up in a new life but once it starts moving, it keeps going if you endure it bit by bit. Like a boulder at the top of a hill that starts rolling down, there comes a time when it will pick up speed and make its own progress and all you need to do is keep its route clear of obstacles. A lot needs to be considered and because of my health, I had my work cut out, but nothing is impossible if the right changes are made to serve as a structure that holds work together.

Perhaps my health was a blessing in disguise and realising this is so helpful because it is a challenge and with that comes the self-compulsion to keep going. I try to see it this way and it helps me put my old life behind me and make the stretch because I know why I am continuing. There are useful things I can take from my old life and mould into my new life and the second I start this is when the new life begins. If I like I can think of the whole thing as a project and use my skills to progress and make something I want for myself. I now have a lot that has been through my head, and I need to use this more than ever now. Looking back, there was a certain amount of flippancy in my attitude, as if I was trying to be able to do nothing more than have fun when I should have been persevering with a sensible routine. My original ideas were not grounded on living a long happy time, which does involve some work, and is what we should all want and work for. I am trying to not lose the plot and stay on a good path.

Nowadays, I don't worry if I oversleep or need to give myself a notification that I want a day off anymore. I do what I need to do, and nobody can say anything about it, but I am keeping it sensible. I oversee how many breaks I take and how long they are, and due to my health, I am generous. I get my work done for me and this is a happy place to be. The important work I do is for my own good and that is what I try to focus on. After moulding a plan together, it was time to act and not put down roots. I cannot spend too much time planning this change in life and not enough time implementing it. It is such a big change that I must consider there will always be changes going on here and there. So, I start with the big changes and then get stuck into the work, and then I can start thinking that I am not going to waste time. MS is the catalyst that has brought about a change, and I need to sort that out. I did work with MS for years and years and gained support from the government to do so and I am thankful and know that I could get support if I went to a job. The work I put in place was more born out of my life experiences that were right and proven. Trust me, my time will still be wasted as I am trying to focus on using it for good, not letting it slip past unused. I must use these opportunities and not dismiss them. I am going with the opportunities as they come and seem to whittle down to one workload. There may be missed opportunities passing me by and I can't take them all at once. Never mind.

I have done things on my own before, but they were always done alongside a job and employment was in place. This time, I have started completely on my own and I have the experience to help me do it. If it concerns my health, then that will need to be included in the work. I am including a heavy presence of workouts and exercise in the scheme I am following because of my health condition, and this would not be possible with a job. I can't see even the most liberal employer allowing me to meditate for half an hour during the day. I am pretty sure the other employees would have something to say about that being unfair. I never spent much time focusing on my fitness and I am thankful I can now incorporate this into my work in a healthy way. I would be doing exercises in my spare time if I was employed and that would take it out of me so maybe this is the way forward for people with health issues, and who knows, it may be a big success in my health. I really think this is worth a shot. Basically, if I can find the time to exercise and work on a new life, I am sure it is best for me, so if I can't accommodate that alongside a conventional job then so be it. I must try different things and make what works stick. The way I used to try and fit everything in was silly because it was too much. My life was too busy and I lacked time to meditate and read the Bible and these are very dear to me. So, the way everything is changing from my old way is better for me and I will maintain it and not put so much time into work and more into health and well-being. I will no longer attempt to get more out of something that is hopeless. The past has taught me enough to create a more suitable future.

It was time to be brutal and totally remove the practices in my life that were not beneficial, even if they were things that I had done all my life. I am fully aware of what a calamity my life was and would be if things didn't change and so I was ruthless. Yes, being diagnosed with MS is what it took to change and that is what it needed, but it is good exercise anyway, regardless of health. I needed something that would shake me down to the core but not kill me or leave me without a chance of redemption. There was too much in my life that I had given value to for one reason or another, whereas the only thing of importance is me. It is as if I was surrounding myself with distractions when all I needed was to focus on a rewarding life. The whole exercise was useful to get me out of a bad life that was pointless and it gave me an understanding of the possibilities I could find and work with. My mind was open to being a person who wants to enjoy life without needing material items to do this. Marketing no longer had a hold and thinking about what other people were doing was not so important.

It is as simple as this: I know what I need to do and how I need to do it and so must find the drive and compulsion needed to do it. I will carry out this task and get as far through it as possible. I may tweak it over the years to improve it if I don't lose my way. It is important that I keep mindful of this endeavour and don't get distracted or risk everything I have become for simple pleasures. I am at a point where I don't have anything to lose, but if that changes, then it may be problematic to keep the direction I am on and so I will need prayer and meditation more than ever.

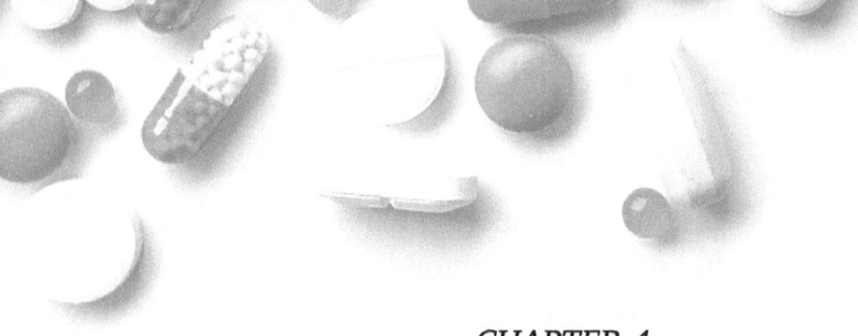

CHAPTER 4

A start to a new way of life

When life got real, it showed me who wasn't interested and offered me time to work out what my options were. It is important for a person to understand that things change in life, and it will happen eventually to most people whether they want it to or not. It was important that I took steps to deal with the change in my life and didn't allow it to get out of my control. I understand that what happened to me was not the end, but if I played my cards right, it could be the beginning of something. It is sometimes hard to be prepared for all trials, but this gave me a new purpose. I discovered my survival instinct. When there is a big change of some sort, it is going to have a knock-on effect on your situation and abilities, depending on the type of change. For me, it was the start of everything in my life taking a new direction. Don't panic if you no longer fit in because it is okay to stand out. You will find you fit in elsewhere and that might call for a move in your situation no matter how long you have been in it. Keep working on letting go of the old life and building a new life; it is so refreshing. Because of my situation, I am no longer trying to achieve my old goals and have started to set new ones. There is always a more suitable way to live and getting as close to this state is where the work is needed. I know it involves health and well-being, so this is going to be a major part of my new life and I am okay with that. To be honest, it should have always been an important part.

I think a routine is essential in knowing where you are in terms of activities undertaken, and this was a good place for me to start. I don't want to miss out on taking my medication or anything else of importance and so this is going to be a part of my routine for sure. Following a well-thought-out routine will soon become ingrained in my mind and the important parts of it will become like the foundations. It will take time and energy to get fully set into a new life, so I am giving it a chance to settle in, and not rushing it will help to make it as good as possible. I want direction and tasks to be a normal part of my life which is going to take a bit of care in setting up and I will be doing all this from scratch. Therefore, it is important to start on the key things and then add other items while maintaining the most important foundations like exercise and medication. There are going to be things I need to keep working on so I need a healthy attitude that will stop me from quitting because I understand its importance. The idea I have is to try not to ever give up on myself and my condition, and instead, build a life that does not just revolve around my health. The time is needed, and so I am taking it one step at a time but am sure all things can be achieved. I can find no fault in trying and plenty in not.

I could see this need coming for a long time and so was considering it up front and got myself prepared. I knew the life I was living was not going to benefit my health and, at some time, it needed to change otherwise it would leave me with a greater challenge. The MS thing is what was going to happen to me and was not going to be easy and you may understand, therefore, why I put off making changes in my situation while I could. Am I now prepared to adjust and do what I need to even if it takes years? Back then, it was a state of knowing what was coming and what I needed to do about it. I think this shows character that although things had changed, a person does not give up trying to do something with their time.

I was needing to commit to it even though there were going to be times when I wanted to quit, and I needed to get past them. Staying focused on the journey is the attitude I use, and the time is here and now. It is important to find something to do and, even if it involves you changing a career and learning a new skill, then don't be afraid of the challenge. Enjoy the fact that you have time to really understand yourself and have spent time learning as much as possible. What has changed in my life is huge and not through choice and I have seen the improvement in my life that I still need to achieve, God willing. I have made sacrifices, and to be honest, I have not made sacrifices in what matters in the way of my old life being changed just to benefit my health. I have made a few mistakes too and learned a few lessons as a result which is okay because I am not perfect, and I learned that the mistakes were occurring because of lack of experience and doing something original.

All in all, MS is a lifelong condition and I have kept this as a reminder to keep it real and important. It is hard not to think about it all at one time and so much easier if it can be broken into pieces. What I am doing about it is of the utmost importance, and this has given me the drive to progress with a routine and new skills. I understand that it is all about me and most people are interested in their own situations. So, why have I decided to live like this? And how can I keep it up? These are good things to work out no matter who you are. I can separate myself from certain lifestyles and not feel upset because I know there is this to do. It is all going to build a healthier life. Why would anybody choose a life of ruin? We all have a choice and time to make it.

Just to be clear, historically, I went for years with no real health issues, and then it began to happen so slowly that for ages, I didn't even feel that there was a problem. Any time before an actual diagnosis is an estimation for the exact start of getting MS, but in the beginning, my illness was little and ad hoc yet somewhat noticeable subconsciously, and without realising, I was inadvertently making small changes in which eye or hand I was using when reading and holding things. I didn't know I was ill or when it had begun. It seemed like as far back as I could remember, I'd had a tremble in my right hand, and it went undiagnosed for a long time, but something was changing in me constantly. Them is the breaks. I remember being twenty years old when it started to become an occasional problem and that there was something noticeably and slightly amiss. For starters, I would be holding a cup of tea or coffee when my hand would start to tremble, and I would spill the contents or need to put the cup down. When this would happen, I thought that the problem would pass with time, and I just adjusted my movements to accommodate these issues. I didn't think it would get worse or stay the same and I would continue to adjust my ways to deal with it. I was young and my mind was on other things and so didn't give it any serious thought. These problems wouldn't happen much anyway so they would pass and I would forget about them.

This still happens today, and accidents do happen, only now they happen more often and I know why. I am not thinking that I should have acted sooner because I can't go back - I am more interested in where it goes from here and how to do something going forward. Just imagine it gets more lasting and affects my eating so that I get the food or drink all down myself daily. If I don't try to do something, I will need serious help. Some days are getting very difficult, and I find myself cleaning up a lot. This is because Nowadays, the times when it doesn't happen are more common. I couldn't go on like that and there came a time to seek help. Even though it sometimes got noticed by friends and family, they never suggested I needed help or recommended seeing a doctor. I guess the average person is not interested in their neighbours as far as helping them and more how they can receive the help. It was during this time that I was making a start to change my life to improve the health of my mind and body. I guess I felt I needed to change my lifestyle and the start of a new life was taking shape. The seed was planted and would grow if cared for.

Now, there are so many times when I have forgotten to take things slow and paid the price, or not fully considered what is involved in actions like going out for a walk. Maybe, on occasions, I am not thinking about my situation properly and I need to take things a bit more slowly to stop myself from making these mistakes. I have tripped and fallen or bumped into stuff many times and this seems to be a hard lesson for me because I keep needing to relearn it. However, don't we all have accidents from time to time? The penny was taking a long time to drop - or maybe I just was being ignorant and didn't want changes in certain ways. I was alone with my problems and played them down a lot when I could have sought help and started off with the medical support that is available. Maybe a person smarter than me wouldn't put up with as much as me and try to live with it as I did and instead seek advice sooner. 4Spending my time learning to live with problems was becoming my life and I either saw no reason to change or wasn't ready to change.

I also developed a condition with my eyesight called nystagmus, which is involuntary eye movements, so I just used one eye mostly and didn't take it seriously. Again, it took years to develop, and this was the one symptom that led me to the diagnosis. When my eyesight problems were developing, I had regular appointments with the opticians, and I just put up with it and didn't even realise that it could be the start of something sinister like MS. I wear eyeglasses and regular eye tests are part and parcel so there was an opportunity there to get help and advice. I remember an optician giving me a letter to give to my doctors after taking a routine eye test. It led to a referral to the hospital ophthalmology department, and I had regular appointments for some time before being discharged with no diagnosis. The same thing happened again, and this time, I was referred to a neurologist as well. I attended many appointments with a growing number of medical professionals. It can be said that the trouble I was having with my eyesight led to my being diagnosed and shows how eyesight can tell a lot about a person's health.

The problem with my eyesight makes it difficult for me to see and this has deteriorated a lot over time. Now that I know about exercising the eyes, I try to practise this regularly, even by moving my eyes rhythmically in different directions as a workout. Sometimes I have a bad day and it's important to be positive and keep going and use the tools available like adjusting screen and font sizes.

It takes time for something like MS to become apparent so it is equally long before the likes of me take it as real. Over the years, my symptoms got slowly worse until it was picked up by my opticians and doctors and so it was a neurologist who made the diagnosis because they are knowledgeable of this. When I was told my diagnosis was MS, I felt the bottom fall out of my world and kept it to myself for weeks. I understand from research that it is important to be diagnosed in good time and there are lots of reasons for other illnesses that cause similar problems to be ruled out first. If people I tell about my condition are thinking as I used to, they might be imagining that I will end up in a wheelchair and having to be cared for. I thought of the worse scenario and that didn't help me one bit. Fortunately, there is information available and if you use it and make the necessary changes, you can carry on living life and enjoying it. The best thing to do is to take time and think about what needs to be done because as soon as you tell unqualified people, they will start filling your head with nonsense. I now know from experience more than I did about MS and how best to handle it. There is a great deal I don't know, and this is a good thing so far as I am putting together an understanding that is unique to me. I can take facts and ideas regarding MS and connect them together to my benefit. If a person is willing, then they can rearrange their affairs and carry on living as they were if they want.

At first, after my diagnosis, I felt confident that I could work and carried on working six days a week for two companies for several years. My health was being treated with medication and I was okay apart from some side effects and one of my eyes going off to the side a lot. There are four main types of MS and I have relapsing-remitting MS which is the most common. This means it is active or dormant and so not always damaging my nerves. The thing is, I very slowly got worse. With MS, no two cases are the same, so I needed to find out my specifics and then make something of myself and my future. For me, I need to take my medication and that is important, and I will be developing a healthy routine to coincide with this. The way I first thought of things was so out of date that it didn't take into account the differences in understanding from decades of advancements and how understanding has grown. It has been decades and I am still nowhere near that bad and that may be partly because I train my body to help improve my coping mechanism. In my case, MS is more dormant than active and this would possibly explain the slow deterioration. I am not making excuses and will continue my routine though because I like it. If I need to take a break and have some water or a lie-down, then that is okay and allowed and is part of exercising. I think the slow rate of deterioration is an opportunity for me to increase my body's power and I am working towards being as well as possible. Don't squander a chance to get ahead in the game so I'm using my time well and this is important. I don't know what tomorrow will bring so I am taking my chance to mend the roof while the sun shines. I never thought it was going to be easy. I had taken an interest in exercising in my life and was able to use this in my daily plan to use exercise to help my body cope with MS. Taking as much time as I want to achieve the best results is fine and fits into the situation I am now in. My life changed and I was able to change too.

The idea I have is to fight to keep MS from taking me over and I am mindful of the problems that have developed so I work on overcoming them. So, I research and study ways to combat MS because this is a useful way to spend time. I don't want to just sit around and give up. Most of my time is available for me to work on my health, so it is silly not to do this because it does make a difference. I guess I am doing what works best so, at the end of the day, I can say that at least I tried and have no regrets. There are other things being done to help and I am playing my part with the spare time I have available. As I find that I have more time to spend, I spend it wisely. I am using my spare time mainly to meditate and pray as well as making sure I eat a healthy diet. My hope is to regain control of my health and not lose any more function, or even just keeping at bay and stabilizing the illness. I am trying everything I can to stop further deterioration and if all I achieve is to slow it down, then I think this is something to celebrate. I've worked out what I want to achieve and how to achieve it and hopefully, there won't be too much disruption. One positive aspect is that I am not seriously affected by my condition and lead a normal life to the best of my ability and am happy. Since time is of the essence with a set routine of medication and treatments, being organized is so important.

Before diagnosis, my diet was not always the best either and so I am making the effort to eat more fruit and veg every day. I had smoked cigarettes for ten years in the past, so considering how my body had been impacted, I had to do some research into improving things. Firstly, I tried to fix an exercise routine and avoid cigarettes ever being around me again and the ban on smoking indoors was a great help. I remember it took years to quit smoking and how expensive it was to buy cigarettes anyway. To quit, I tried chewing gum and cutting down and then, after ten years, only going cold turkey worked for me. I don't think I will smoke anymore, and it is important to be this way for good and so I will need to remember this. I must keep the exercise routine realistic and regular as part of a new life and must always do what I can even if sometimes it is difficult. The only thing I have complete control over is my body and so any part of my routine from exercise to diet is totally my responsibility and will give me some added control over the onset of the illness. Everything I do does get easier over time and that gives me satisfaction and keeps me going as opposed to how I would feel if everything got harder. If things are getting worse, then something needs to change, and I must do the necessary and assess the work I am doing that may need to be changed or improved. It may be a lack of fluid or rest and not forgetting the importance of breathing well. Therefore, I start each day with plenty of fluid in me and maintain my hydration from then on. As for my breathing, I should be taking deep rhythmic breaths – something else to watch out for.

I have programmed my mind to work out regularly and this involves working out even when I don't feel like it. I just do it without thinking and in the best way I can. Exercising regularly is good for my appetite too so I can eat well with lots of fruit and veg and bread because exercising needs fuel. Food provides the body with energy and the energy is needed to progress in my exercises, building strength and stamina. I do not let time spent exercising take anything from my normal life like the ability to clean or cook due to tiredness which is also very important. I, therefore, eat and drink well and this is a by-product of exercise, which is all good. Basically, it all ties together nicely and it seems the more healthy activities I have, the more are added by me for supporting them. When I watch what I eat and drink, then regular exercise doesn't wipe me out and this is the basis of an exercise routine. The only thing left is joy and peace and that can be achieved with prayer and meditation.

Giving time to all these things and seeing the importance of maintaining them means I feel satisfied at the end of each day that I am doing everything in my control. I understand that things happen, and it is not always possible to follow a routine completely every day. For example, if I am ill due to a virus, I will rest and recover and then I must return to my routine of exercise and diet, and still, I can make use of the downtime when I am not able to exercise and I have still got time for prayer and meditation so it is not a total loss. I make sure that any interruptions in my routine are just temporary. Restarting my routine is important after an interruption as there is a risk that I may fall into a trap if I don't, and this is not what I want. There was a time when I stopped driving cars and started taking the bus instead. Then, while I was crossing the road, I was hit by a car during the journey and suffered a broken tibia and fibula due to a reckless driver.

Well, that involved an operation to put a pin in my leg and this was serious so needed a lot of downtime for recovery. It reduced me to no exercise except slightly while I recovered but after I had regained mobility, I restarted my routine in part by doing push-ups and always praying and meditating. Sometimes I pick up a virus and find myself with a temperature and spend the day lying in bed with headaches and just drinking tea, which isn't as serious as a broken leg but still needs downtime. Although I recover, it often leaves me weak which is like a move backwards from where I was in exercises, and I need to regain my strength and stamina. Still, I do as much exercise as I can, and, through a routine, get back to normal the best way I can. Something is better than nothing and at times like these, I need to pray to ask for mental help to get through these trials.

Whether you are well or in a position like me, you should exercise, so keep moving forward and don't give in to a life of laziness. I learned this fact at school and every week had physical exercise (PE) as part of my education and this was not to ever be stopped. After leaving school, it is easy to think you don't need to do PE anymore, but you need to understand it is for your own good and put time aside to do something physical regularly. At first, I weight-trained and ran, and over time, this has become impossible because of the impact of MS on me but if I can't do this thing, I will find something else physical. The important thing is I adapted my exercise routine to fit my circumstances.

MS meant I needed to adjust my routine and I use an exercise bike for 20 minutes twice a week now as a part of my routine instead of running. So, this way, I can maintain a level of cardiovascular training. After a session on the bike, I will need time to recover because it kills my strength and especially in my legs which means I am at risk of an accident if I don't sit down. Recovery involves a stretch of my limbs and lots of cold coffee in my case, but you do what you need to do. I love coffee so much and use it to help me rehydrate and it is mostly water anyway. The number of times I have climbed off the exercise bike and fallen over is a lot but I now know how to fall and land safely, and I know this is an oxymoron, so life isn't without a sense of irony. Due to the increasing time I spend on the bike and the resistance from the pedals, I can become very tired after a session and quite often have to have a chair next to the bike to rest on.

Every day, I use an exercise tower for pull-ups, dips, etc. too and this is a good part of my routine. I spend about one hour a day, spread out, working out on the power tower which is helping my strength increase and I am better when the weather gets cooler too. I have become efficient at using my body mass in exercise. It's the way I can ensure that I can exercise, and I can work out without any equipment if need be. Take push-ups and sit-ups, for example; I can do these anywhere or time without any equipment. I am constantly finding solutions to problems that may not happen often, but if they do, I am ready. Over the years, I have broken multi gyms that aren't cheap, and the solution was to get an exercise tower instead. It is important to be safe and make sure the exercises aren't dangerous. Everything I do is under my control, and this has come with experience and at a price. I know my exercise limitations and don't get carried away or overdo it. All I do is within my ability and at no time am I at risk, so the advice I give is to work out what is suitable for you and don't think you must copy anyone. Only when exercises become easier do I increase the work involved. It has taken time and accidents to ensure a suitable workout and I am always aware of my limitations because they may change for one reason or another. Over time, I have become stronger and that is what happens as a by-product of regular exercise so there is a benefit to doing it. I hold positions in exercises for longer as I get stronger to improve things like coordination and stamina. I don't force anything because there is a likely consequence of having accidents. This is the deal for me, and I have found it out for myself and without a trainer. I can work out and exercise off my own back and this hasn't been easy. I have had accidents and they show I need to concentrate all the time.

On one occasion, I managed to fall awkwardly and break five ribs. I wasn't even working out when this happened but was not thinking about the things I was doing and this is what can happen accidentally. I try to be patient because some things are going to take time, but I am also reaping the benefits of staying with my routine, so I have become thankful for the persistent attitude I have. If I give up, I have admitted defeat and am accepting the problems I have are going to better me. Well, that won't do for me. Anything is possible. Try, try, and try again.

Hydration and food are of the utmost importance. I didn't always do this and, to be honest, I have sometimes spent all morning lacking enough fluids. Now, I drink around a litre of fluid before midday, and this is an example of how you need to pay attention to the body and learn as you go. It may not go to plan with every aspect of a routine and that is okay, so if it isn't happening all the time, maybe that means something needs to be changed and there is always a solution. Think about what is being done.

The emotional effect of my changes has been eye-opening and eye-watering and left me with a feeling of uselessness, so I need to dig deep to cope with it all. It has given me a new purpose in life, and I hope it is a proper calling and not a five-minute wonder and the actions I take will stick. Sometimes I get upset and even though I hold it together, it will mean I take it out on other people, and I am not happy with this. I feel a new start is called for because I have lost everything and all I can do now is start from the beginning although with an MS hindrance. I Have now turned my affairs over, will not give up and will continue to push to the end. It is still me but a new me with a new purpose and a new drive. I have needed to set goals and I am dealing with a life that I need to be managing the best I can with lots of things happening. There is no more being told what to do except for advice from my medical team and everything to do with my health and not giving in to MS boils down to my choices. I need to tell myself what to do and do it which is using motivation and not forgetting the importance of inclusion with treatment for MS. It is one thing to serve somebody and entirely different to serve yourself completely. I need to make the right moves and do my best to suffer as small a loss as possible. I am not ill enough to be looked after and that is good for me, so I want to keep it like that and that is what I am trying to do. It is a case of struggle toward success. The MS makes it my choice one moment, then takes that responsibility away at the next moment. Basically, I work for myself until the strategy is well established, and then I am working for that. It comes down to whom I obey. First, I obey our heavenly Father, and after that, I am working toward a normal life, and this comes down to me and then itself. I need to be sensible and make sure I rest and exercise while making sure I take food and fluids on board and so I am trying to put together a timetable to follow as guidance. I cannot just do a simple routine that takes care of things, so I am putting my heart into one and changing who I am. There are important parts of my life I follow and stick to, and I do leave myself spare time as well so I can relax and entertain myself. When it comes down to it, I am moving in a direction that I must maintain and transform myself into a new way of thinking and behaving if this is going to work.

Due to the fact I have MS, I have spent a huge amount of time working out the best course of action to keep it under control and this can be a full-time job. I have been studying and talking about MS with everyone I can while trying to keep myself fit for purpose. The purpose is to live an ordinary life. My definition of ordinary life is unique to me. It would have been so much easier if a full day-to-day action plan was available, but sadly, there isn't because everyone is unique so will need to find their own way to best suit them. Since we are all different in stature and age, I could not find one action plan to suit me and deal with the type of MS I have but the basics are there. The best chance I have is to set up a routine focused on medication and exercise. So, here I am living a life that I have designed; a life that leaves me some time to enjoy myself, and an equal amount to address my problems. There is always going to be time to work out and there is always going to be spare time to enjoy myself and do other things. I do the best I can, and it is all a regular part and a very important part of surviving. We are imperfect in lots of ways but can work on them if we want. There are lots of things that can go wrong with the body, and likewise, ways to deal with them, and it can take something like MS to give someone the motivation to use their lifestyle as a part of treatment alongside their medicine. A healthy lifestyle works and, alongside medicine, will improve things and keep me going in a satisfactory way. I am not saying that my lifestyle is to blame for my health problems; quite the opposite - it can improve my health and should be used in this way. I would not have been able to achieve much on my own and remain thankful for the support I receive. I have given up on so much and become something else due to my health giving me a job to get on with. Although the treatment and exercises suitable for me may not suit everyone else, at least I might be able to show others that there is a way to help yourself, and being able to help others deal with their issues is very important.

The life I lead has gone through a change and I have had to metamorphose into a different person due to being diagnosed with MS. Is this process of metamorphosis something that we all do in our lives, I wonder? When I consider a person then I can understand that we carry on changing all through life and this is what we all do. I need to think about the cycle of life to fully get my head around this. I need to think about what I am going through and focus on this being a stage that is changing me from the core into a new life. So, I am in a state of change and the product remains to be seen. The important thing is that I know that physically and emotionally, I can influence my change. The most important thing I can do is keep making good new decisions and changes to benefit myself. Life is a gift from our heavenly Father. This is the most precious and amazing gift and therefore something worth looking after. Even if life is not easy and gets damaged along the way, there is still a good reason to take the best care of oneself and advances in medicine and fitness are all in support of this. I cannot replace my life with a different one and it is not a possession that can be treated without respect. So, try your best to live a good life even if things get tough at times. Just keep reminding yourself that there is work to be done and be at peace with everything.

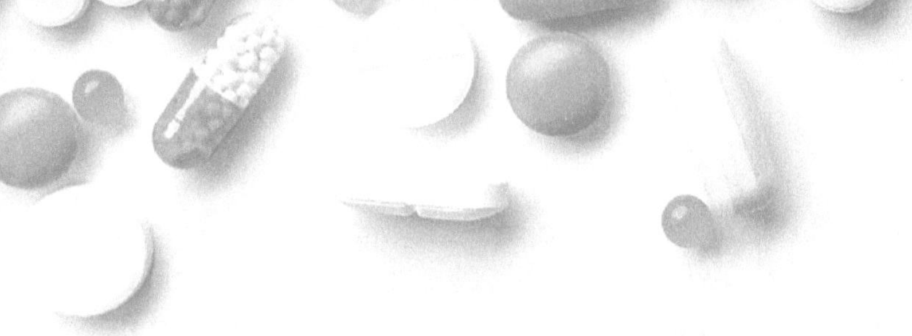

CHAPTER 5

The weird understanding of people

It is important to be careful how we speak about other people as each day may bring circumstances that affect their lives and their reactions. If a person is having a bad day, they may not be able to react to you in the same way as they would on a good day. A person may also be associated with others who share their opinions with them and that can become the way that person also thinks because they want to fit in with these associations. I am no fan of some of the treatments I have been subjected to from people over the years since my symptoms have become visible and They could have acted in that way for many reasons. Often things are said as a joke when, in actual fact, their comments can hurt I could take it up with that person purely to find peace but tend to only do that if it becomes a regular occurrence. Sometimes people have no interest in anyone but themselves and I accept this, but I am surprised about my own family at times and their lack of trying or empathy. I mean, when your own blood turns away, it leaves you feeling at rock bottom. Of course, I may just be being paranoid and be totally wrong in how I think about my family's behaviour because *I* am having a bad day and am taking it out on them as we all do. I think that everyone needs to stop and think a bit more and not react too fast.

When I was first diagnosed, everyone wanted to help me, and, over the years, acquaintances and friends and family have gradually distanced themselves from me. I think that they want to get on with things and feel I affect this in some way. It feels as if they are bored with me no longer fitting in the way I did and now see me as a burden because it is lasting longer than they thought it would. I don't understand what people who know me think is going to happen. Well, the thing is, MS is a lifelong condition and they must have decided they are okay with never seeing me again. From his actions, for example, I am inclined to feel that my father thinks of my brother as everything and me as nothing, and so I need to brush that off because I don't know for sure. I am probably entirely wrong. People are more interested in how they are perceived themselves and even though this is not right, it is not against the law and so I live with it. The important thing is to maintain myself and forget about other people sometimes. It needs to be said that I don't want people to think they need to care for me but if they want me to go out with them, they could ask me how they can help like what I can do and where I want to go instead of just asking me if I want to do what they are doing. Sometimes I think people look at the negatives and what the effects are and don't think about what a person can still achieve. If friends want to go out as a group, then I may not be willing to join in with it, but that doesn't mean they can't see me in some other way. When people dislike you, they want everybody else to dislike you too and then the lies begin. There may be a person who knows you and doesn't want anyone else to know you. In Ecclesiastes 7:9, we learn to keep our temper under control; it's foolish to harbour a grudge. This advice is what I need to use a lot, but this may be because I have changed since getting MS. Do they not care what I think of them? Really, I only care what Jehovah thinks and it is not worthwhile getting anxious about people's behaviour. I will need to face and embrace my difficulties or risk them affecting my mental health. I want to keep my dignity.

I know from comments that I've overheard that some people thought I was drunk when I was out and about and they saw my movements, but it doesn't hurt to ask if I'm okay instead of making assumptions. That way, they may have learned something about how to be caring towards others. I think differently about this because my condition now causes these situations. I am what I am and maybe a bit biased, but this is a good opportunity to help others with understanding MS and other conditions. I can't tell everyone about my situation, and I need to consider that not everyone has the spare time and so I think the best idea is to write about it. I can't expect everyone to understand all the ins and outs of MS anyway, especially if it doesn't affect them or anyone they care about. I only know about MS in some depth myself because I have it and it is always on my mind. My issue is with those who find out about me and show no sympathy and feel it's an issue they want someone else to deal with. I can only imagine if they got MS how they would feel. I think maybe I should think about the person MS has made me into. Do I think MS is an issue someone else should deal with? Also, if a person goes further and uses the information against me then they are a low life, and I should avoid them. In the Dickensian way, they are nasty. If having MS interferes with somebody else's life and so they actively do me wrong and treat me unfairly or differently to bully me, it is wrong and there is no reason for it. I think the problem you see is that I am going to be distanced from everyone eventually. I would not want to make someone with MS feel worse about their illness, so why can't friends just do something with me on a different occasion – something I can enjoy and join in with? Does society leave us all pigeonholed when it should bring us all together? I look forward to a time when there is no sickness.

When my condition became known to my friends, acquaintances and family, that was when the assumptions began because people all seem to think they know everything about MS and have a thing or two to say as a result. Now, I may be a bit aggressive when I talk to some people, and it may be frowned upon, yet people have said horrible things to me but in a nice calm way and they get away with it because of this, yet I am the one to get in trouble when it upsets me and I raise my voice to them. It is often what is said and not how it is said that needs understanding. I'm sure most people have heard of MS and don't dispute they know of somebody who is suffering from it and that is where it should stop. My medical team only talks about what I am going through with me and never what is to become of me because they don't know, and they are professionals. I have been told by friends and acquaintances of ways to treat MS that don't exist or make no sense and it makes me wonder why the person doesn't just talk about the weather or maybe sport instead. If the person has an interest, then they should stick to questions and l will be happy to tell them how I am and all about MS from my health experience. Does it hurt to ask how I am? It is as if some of my friends have been on the internet and spent five minutes reading a page and now think they can give advice when I have a medical team for that and so don't need advice from them. I am sure most people don't know much else than the basics and are just aware of MS and don't even know the medications now available. It took years for me to learn what I have and what the impact is but eventually, people I knew started to pick up on everything about me and it felt like there were some who would use it against me.

We all make mistakes and just because I have MS doesn't mean my mistakes are caused by that. Rather than spending time with me and asking questions on my particular path, they seem to focus on what I cannot do and stop giving me a chance to even try, and this happened especially at work. Why nobody asked me is odd and I can't figure that out. Often, the argument they had was time-based and not relevant. Someone should have asked me questions from time to time but failed to talk to me about it properly and made assumptions a lot when instead, I was quite happy, to tell the truth, and how things can change for the better otherwise people should think about something else to discuss. Has nobody got time these days? I felt that everyone was watching my every move at work and using this information in some way to decide what I should be doing. Currently, I know that I could get support, however, some people in my life became hurtful, and I felt so low that they should be ashamed of themselves. If someone is ill, they need to see a professional and get advice, not a friend or acquaintance. If you want to help them, then tell them that they should see a professional and see how they get on. It may be more serious than is realised and not being treated may cause more harm than good. I've had injuries caused by sports and exercise wrongly interpreted by people because they know I have MS and thankfully, in the end, I have seen a professional and received the correct treatment. I think it is important to realise there is a difference between a person giving their opinion and a person with experience and knowledge treating me.

Some people have made me feel very low at times by not talking to me about my health but listening to their friends regarding me instead. It seemed people thought I was unable to benefit others and should stay at home on benefits where I would be forgotten. Was this a form of discrimination or hate? My illness became who I was, and it took a lot for me to feel that, even with my issues, I still had a lot to offer. People looked at me as having MS first and that is discrimination because it is important to understand the person as well and see they are separate. It was like my issues walked into a room before me and everybody had already made an opinion and formed preconceptions before I even walked into the room. My work colleagues started saying things about MS that showed a lack of kindness and it became obvious to me that they saw me as a liability. People I was introduced to had first been told that I had MS which I felt would have been better coming from me. Sometimes I struggle and sometimes I don't and there can be various factors that affect me. Even my employer started treating me with a lack of generosity and it was because, in their heads, they had a list of things I couldn't do and that it was only going to become worse. This didn't happen overnight but gradually over years, and I regret nothing because look at what I have gained and the opportunities I have now as a result. I now have the idea to create something new from nothing which is wonderful. Here is an idea... rather than thinking about what I can't do, look at what I can do! On occasions, as if to validate their opinion, people would say they were friends with a doctor. This may be true and if a doctor was talking about me to other people without seeing my records or me to other people then they are breaking the law. A qualified doctor knows this and therefore it wouldn't happen. Offering me the wrong support shows ignorance and forcing it on me is a crime. If I need help, I will ask and don't need to be told so. I don't want unneeded help forced on me because it is a depressing and irritating action. All that is needed is the kindness to give help to someone who asks for help in the way they want and not the other way around. The inconvenience to the person who is helping will be small compared to the feelings they get. I am talking about the love that you feel when you care for someone's needs more than your own and the feeling it gives you. The Bible teaches us first to love Jehovah and then to do unto others as ourselves. I wish everyone felt like this.

At work, the treatment people used toward me was getting less caring and this was growing as if there was something sinister happening behind my back. I felt like I was getting in the way, and it would be better if I wasn't there because they didn't need me. Everything I was going through was getting in the way of my thinking and that was unhealthy, and it was time to make a change. Work went into shifts, and I didn't want to choose an option and throw my lifestyle in the bin. I didn't want to be left trying to recover from a workout at work rather than at home in my bed.

There are opportunities like this in life and you need to seize them and, even if they are as daunting as moving house, take them. I am no longer living my life to be as comfortable as I can and that is a great thing because I need to be alert again. I am not suggesting that being too comfortable is bad, but it is not the best way to be and there must be some activities that are pushing me out of my comfort zone which is healthier. When I woke up in the morning, I wanted purpose and was not getting it going to work for the same man every day. To change, I needed to make sacrifices and possibly major ones, so I just stepped away from caring about my work and that did the trick. Firstly, I separated myself from what my life had become, which can be a scary and unknown process. Everything about me was mundane and boring, so I needed a fresh start, and this took time to put in place. I must have spent a year or so thinking about anything I could but there was a pandemic going on, so I needed to stay inside anyway. I was fed up with just existing and craved a challenge that would take up my whole time. To start, I kept fit and, at times, I found the Bible invaluable and so am working on my health and faith. I now understand that with a new life, I was going to become something else and better, but only if I put in the effort. I think MS is just a condition that can be managed among everything else and so I aim to do just that. I do know that no two cases are the same which means no two ways of managing them are either and so my routine is tailored specifically to me which means more work. Most people show compassion, and these are the people I need to be around so it is important to have good people and not bad people to socialise with or you will risk gaining bad habits. It is not difficult to distance people who have a negative outlook anyway. It may not be intentional, but some people want to push me into panicking over my illness, however, I am the expert on me and so I need an element of self-control.

Forgiveness for all things is not the easiest to feel and can take time. However, it is essential so give it time and let yourself escape the feelings of unforgiveness. I don't want to go through life thinking that people are bad because they are just misguided and the last thing I need is to worry myself sick when going out. I can't run the risk of developing an attitude that nobody can be trusted. Most people are good, and I need this knowledge, or I will end up bitter and twisted. There is a chance I will shut myself away from people and I need to fight that urge because there may be times when I need the contact for good reason. I want to live a life of peace and happiness and that will make me free, and even though a person may find it hard to understand the complexities of my health, I don't hold that against them. Having the right attitude is healthy and will benefit me more than the wrong attitude will and so I need to stay positive and acknowledge when I need to rest and not feel bad when I am unable to make the effort. What does it matter what people think anyway? It's just their opinion.

I have enough to worry about and my health is not going to benefit from stress and worry. I need to think about taking my medication and developing a healthy lifestyle and that may not leave room for much else. I want to distance myself from people who are not compassionate, and it is as simple as avoiding thought. There are people who help and support me and some who interfere and want to control me, and they are easily separated. The problem with employers is not going to stop me, and I will succeed in one way or another, and maybe without one. Rome wasn't built in a day, and I will build a new life and leave behind those who hold me back. I need the desire and commitment to do my best; this is what I am working on, and, if I need something to pray about, this is a start and it is going to help because I'm pleasing Jehovah when I turn to him. We must be aware that all that is needed is our best no matter how small it may be. Understand this, though, that what a person sees is not everything to be seen about me. I am seeing what needs to be seen regarding me and the effort I make.

I can do a job and there would be minimal adjustments compared to a person without MS or any other serious problem, and I know this even if nobody else does. When people learn that I have MS, they don't even want to give me the chance to show that I can work. I can understand an employer feeling like this but it does seem unfair. I have not given up on working but instead, if a career change is necessary, then I will do it. It may be that people are of the opinion that everybody needs to be 100 percent to work or maybe they need to be young and I urge a person who thinks this to take a good look in the mirror. This may be true of certain jobs and that's where it should end. There are things that I am better suited to and some jobs that I would struggle to do. There are jobs that I need help in and then there are jobs that I am the best for because they suit me due to the level of impact MS has on me being low. These attitudes that MS is a problem and can't be supported cause me to lose faith in humanity. You see, medication and ways to make work more suitable are far from what they were. If you are looking for somebody with experience in MS, or just nerve damage, then I am very experienced. I can show you the way to a good life with purpose. That is a very unlikely job, and my point is that I may find work that is made for someone like me. I am sure there are employers who know this and believe that I am okay and capable. There are two ways to approach this if someone has MS: You could ask how they are, how long they have had it and what medication they are using to help them cope, or you could only be interested in the problems caused by their illness and ignore all their coping strategies.

It is not responsible to be the best without thinking of others and helping them reach the same level. It is essential to value teamwork and to encourage and help others to reach their potential. Think of equality when thinking of others and not the impact on you or being selfish and wanting everything for yourself. I am an advocate for all those discriminated against in these ways and if I hear someone talk in a negative way about a person's health, I want to educate that person so they see the potential everybody has. I have learned this the hard way and all companies need impartial views when looking at people whom they employ. This does cut both ways and I want employees to do their best too and show that they can work together with all types of people. In the world today, we need each other, and it is important to know this because a person is going to become more dependent for many reasons like age or illness and then the shoe is on the other foot. I don't think it should need to come to this and people should all care about each other without being in a situation that opens their eyes for personal reasons. I now realise the truth that we are the best for each other, and, as diverse as we are, there is a place for everyone, and it is wonderful to see the happiness on offer to all. Therefore, we need to encourage others to think of those less fortunate first with the aim of making them equal.

We are not all the same and we all think differently too. There is that great truth that as a team, we are the best and we can work together, everyone being involved and giving their best when we put our hearts into it. We need to always have this in our minds and drop the attitude of being better off than others both in situations and emotions. Forget about money because all we really need is shelter, clothes and food in our bellies to survive and there is enough for everybody to be satisfied. Sure, it is going to cost money for the basics and that is its use, and it only seems to become a problem when people want more and more. If you can find peace in the basics, you will have more time for others and that is where true happiness is found. Giving is better than receiving.

I love talking and listening to other people when I have spare time because I am very busy surviving, and I don't want to miss out on the company because it is emotionally healthy for everybody. Therefore, I find time to continue with my work to maintain my health and also spend my spare time talking with other people. Conversing should be a part of everyday life and if we all agree to put our differences aside, then it would happen, and we could learn about others and ourselves from this. Communication gives me delight and I want people to see this and copy it and feel delighted also. I may need help and encouragement in some way, and it is worthwhile to talk about this and many other things that are causing me difficulties. It is easy to miss the fact that I have MS because it is internal and without telling them, a person may not know. Sometimes, a person just needs a hand to hold or an ear to listen for some reason and if I lost this connection, I would suffer immensely, and this is what keeps me involved with people. I need these things myself. I find that Jehovah is a great help if I am lonely and surrounding myself with Christians brings me joy and a family of caring people. In Psalm 23, we learn that Jehovah is always with us from when he cares for us to when we are going through dark valleys emotionally. I have been guilty in the past of not putting enough time aside for others and I know this is a sign that I want to change. I have seen the light and it has taken a lot to get me here, but I am helping it grow. I am lucky that I have worked this out and accept that people bring me so much joy. I live with plenty of people all around who only think of what they want, and people just want more and more. More than anything material, my association with Jehovah and fellow Christians brings me more joy than just being around other people. Therefore, I am working on my relationship with Jehovah, and this is a refuge for me when I feel depressed because after all, I am only human and sometimes, when I find myself alone, I pray and am looking for salvation. It is important to remember this because if I forget it, I run a risk of letting everything I am going through get too much. I don't want to end up a lost cause. I want to always see there is a way forward.

There are good people who are selfless and do put their needs before others with greater needs. I enjoy their company a lot and their behaviour is rubbing off on me in the way that I have begun thinking of others as they do. I now find it useful to switch off when surrounded by selfish people, so their behaviour does not rub off on me and corrupt the way I act around others, and I think that I will be enjoying the company of selfless people more. There is more to life than meets the eye and with some, all they think of is what they see and possess. I want to show people that they have equal opportunities and that where there is a will, there is a way and they are free to choose the life they lead. The work I do is to try and show people that just because I have disabilities caused by MS does not mean I have no use. Most of my [spare time is spent supporting and educating people so that they will open their minds up and think about others. I have worked with plenty of people over the years who only seem to ridicule others. The main problem I face is being able to focus on my life from my perspective which involves shutting out people who think I should be focused on positions first and that is why I keep practising how To talk to these people. It is important to be generous with those who need an ear to talk to because it will make them feel better when they don't have this from anyone. I am a grown-up and responsible for myself so I know that if I can't help, I can find someone who can. However, there are things I am unable to achieve alone because I am only human and knowing this is key to successfully being a part of an organization or community. On my own, I will not survive no matter what I can do and so it was important for me to learn that I need others for some things. As far as humanity goes, there needs to be unity among everybody involved. We are trying with laws and principles, but it is not enough because men cannot seem to govern themselves. Without having a reason to try hard, to progress in life with each other is futile. I remember being young and naïve and that only got me so far so now I have a chance to make amends and going forward with this is important and stops me from giving up. Think about how dependent a baby is and then realise that your dependencies may change over time, through age, illness or infirmity, and we will all require the assistance of others during those times.

The last job I had carried on for years and I stuck it out even when other opportunities arose so there must have been good times, but they evaporated as my health deteriorated. I can see a connection between my work opportunities and my health which suggests that there was a level of discrimination present. Over the years before I had been diagnosed, I had become aware of how other people look on disability. Then, as I deteriorated and learned it was MS, I was trying to not take anything personally I don't know for sure, but I got the impression that people would say I was unable to do things even though I was able. I was diagnosed with MS and was upfront with my employer about everything and they supported me somewhat until, for whatever reason, they became callous. I worked at the company from pre- to post-diagnosis and that gave me a full experience of the way people perceived my situation and their unwillingness to see past their own unqualified opinion. I saw first-hand how the company treats people with lifelong illnesses and I am not just talking about myself. It wasn't just me who was treated wrong. I never failed to do my job so I really can't get my head around how some acted towards me, and the things they said about me Having a social event with other employees where drinks were involved certainly loosened the tongues of some people and I was told to my face by other employees that I did nothing and often by people who had no idea of what I did.

Over the years, I saw employees come and go and some of them had lifelong conditions, like epilepsy, for example, which seemed to be the reason they lost their job. This employer was not seen to be doing their best for the employees and it all came across as fishy to me. It seemed the company employed people with problems and then made them leave when the problems became a challenge for the company, which just wanted to make money. To be honest, I am concerned about the company's health and safety doing a poor job and failing the employees. I am sure they need to rethink their obligations to employees before they are sued for breaking the law and maybe get rid of the bad influences who work there and replace them with qualified people rather than the company's friends and family. It stands to reason that the larger they become, then the more they are going to need to restructure the way they do things. Thankfully, this company is not representative of all others, and those that use nepotism, such as my previous company, should be closed down for not treating employees fairly under employment law.

I was happy that I left the company and now have new and exciting things planned. That company had no reason to treat me the way they did when I got MS, but I took as much as I could when they made me redundant to support my new direction. I guess I may have burned any bridges I had there.

Emotionally, it is important to put these things behind me and focus on my future. There is no profit in what happened and only what will happen and the only thing I can take from the former is knowledge and experience. It may have taken some time, but I now have a greater understanding of how an employer must put in place the correct adjustments if they want to employ certain people. I do believe it is beneficial not to take on staff with disabilities and then try to put in place what is needed. That is back to front – make the adjustments and then welcome the employee back.

So, I have an idea of where I want to go from here and I must keep focused on it or lose sight of it. I am sure that I want to be involved with society in some way and will keep this aspect in my life. I am doing things to move into a new career and whatever it takes to carry on. I can continue growing spiritually and this gives me an opportunity to engage with people as a Christian and preach as needed. This is an opportunity to try and find a new direction and I need to go for it. I am giving myself the job of finding a reason to get out of a comfortable life and into a position that is stretching me which is healthy for my mind. It may take time with good days and bad days and in-between days, but c'est la vie. I want to move on with life expecting there are going to be a lot of similarities to my old life and that means I have something in the locker. The obstacle I think I face that is likely to cause the most problems is people's opinions and there are ways to deal with that. One way to deal with this obstacle is to remove it from the equation. When I remove things from my life, it will leave a space and therefore, I will try to fill it up with a more suitable activity. There is no other option for me because I have skills that can be used. I need to be strong and courageous. If someone says something hurtful, I need to rise above it and reason whether they are of any interest to me or not. I must realise that I can't waste my time on critics but I must not hate them because they might have issues they are dealing with, and it is just unfortunate that we have crossed paths at that time. I must learn to give such people and opportunities a second chance.

Opinions will change but that won't happen by itself. It is only a person who has an opinion of MS and those who have life-changing conditions who may show an interest in my success. So, I am focused on my health, and that is where it ends for me, and I am only interested in myself for a reason: I need to move on and then I will be able to see what is available in the future. I don't care what anyone apart from my medical team thinks about my health and I want to be an example of how to fight my health condition and something the team is impressed by. This is not because I only care about myself, but more because I need to commit time to my well-being and focus on it on its own when I can. I will always find time for others in my routine because, without time to share, I will suffer a lot more emotionally than is apparent.

This is a lot for anyone to go through, so I take my time and it is a matter of patience. What with different medications and exercise routines to keep on top of, it is natural to have times when cracks develop. So, the most important thing is to pick yourself up and keep going and disprove all those doubts while proclaiming that anything is possible. If I let it happen, I will end up with nothing to look forward to and that is no good and so I keep trying, again and again, to get through the problems. Getting through the problems is one thing, but I must remain happy too. The least I can do at these times is talk to anyone available and there is always someone who understands and can put my mind at rest. Sleeping on things and seeing how I feel in the morning does help and I always do this rather than acting too fast and risking making mistakes. I have done this in the past and it was not good... all it gave was an understanding of how not to behave. I keep myself busy anyway and I am always too busy to get too depressed. I don't allow myself to get bored and can always find things to do. The right way for me to act is in conjunction with my health. So, I don't pay too much attention to people and what they say except when it comes to my medical team, and I keep busy and sleep over stubborn thoughts. I find the bigger variety of opinions I get, the better I can maintain a neutral opinion. It is like the internet and how algorithms pick up what you view and then send you more of the same - I view a big variety to get a good, rounded understanding of my condition. Basically, I try to talk to as many people as I can about the things I do to help me to cope with MS, and then people who can give advice on MS from their own experiences are drawn to me. It is important to remain open-minded and don't take opinions to heart.

It will never stop amazing me that some people will go out of their way to reinvent the wheel, taking the guidance and knowledge available and then building onto it to gain a setup that has the correct foundation and personal needs added. I mean, why don't some people stick to what they know and freely admit what they don't know? I don't know the first thing about some things and would need to start at the beginning To make anything out of them, but this all takes time so if I want to learn, I need to make time. There isn't even experience on certain items that I can gain without spending some time. Everything is going to need work and time. It worries me to think that some people think they can circumnavigate the effort and time needed to understand MS and come to a correct conclusion on their own thoughts. Maybe it is possible to do this, but it is highly unlikely. Look, I find it bizarre that a person can think that I seem okay until they find out that I have MS and then they start stopping me from activities they think put me at risk. Rather than make assumptions about a person's health, the best course of action is to learn about it. We are all different, and, although there are four main types of MS, there are infinite variations within them.

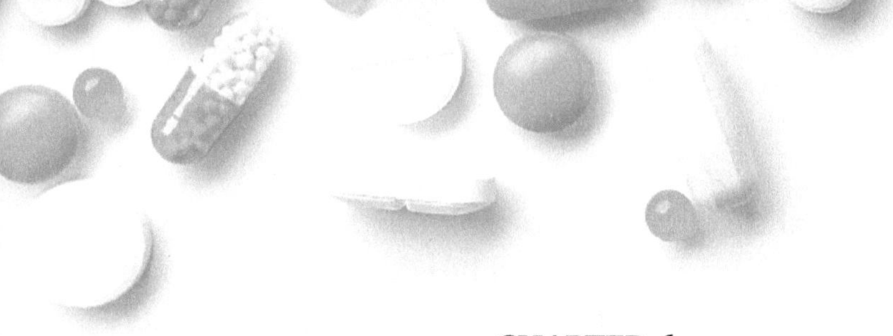

CHAPTER 6

Get into the right state of mind

It is important to realise the challenge is not going to be easy, but you are not alone and what you are doing goes hand in hand with medical research. Tell yourself that no matter how hard it gets, you are going to make it possible to carry on and everything you achieve is worthy of congratulations. It is important to know the fact that my present situation is not my destination and is only part of the journey I am on. I have every chance of leading a good life and I keep telling myself this. I also assure myself that I am going to be okay. I find it hard to keep telling myself this, but I know it will help keep me going even when I feel down. Success is not going to be easy to achieve and I am realistic about it and I keep telling myself this so that I understand it will be hard work but necessary and rewarding. I think of the challenge and not about the time it needs and what is involved because that is an unknown quantity, so instead, I focus on where the challenge is going and what I want to get out of doing it and what to do to achieve this success. If there are some obstacles along the way, then I will do my best to pass them or go around them and even through them. I am up for not letting anything stop me and working hard on making progress which is the key to remaining in control.

Once I have got this straight in my mind, there is only an objective to continue aiming for. Put the effort in. I have seen people who are making the effort in trials, and they are an inspiration to me and something to look out for in society. It is amazing when you learn what the body is capable of and there are plenty of examples to focus on and meditate on. When there is an understanding that there is nothing but a result to reach, then there is a reason to continue.

The job I have put in place is a task that I find best tackled a day at a time. Reflection on how I was going to end up helps me see the job is working. I think of harnessing the body's capabilities and running with it through the struggles. There will be hard times and I may feel the stress and anxiety that goes with them, and I look forward to the good days to come and how I will feel at that time. I don't know what is around the corner or in the future, so all I can do is wake up each day and stay confident. I am positive and open to the changes, whatever forms they take and ignore the idea that it is impossible because I disagree. It is important not to give up but to continue and take it one step at a time.

As far as treatment goes, I leave that to the professionals, although I do follow what they say is healthy very closely. After a while, when the most suitable medication is taken care of and I am settled on it, then I have a lot of time on my hands to work with. I give the medication my trust in this matter and my job is to work on my body for this is completely my responsibility. I am working hard to exercise my body and spirit. I recognise the need to self-train and use personal discipline to try and fulfil my goal. Now and then, I do get feelings that I am wasting my time and I push them aside because I don't have time for negative thinking. It seems to me those feelings are caused by a lack of food or hydration anyway, so this is where it is important to remember that I have dedicated myself to a routine and should focus on it and not ways out of doing it. It is very important to ignore those negative thoughts because they will trap and snare me, and I may end up doing nothing. It is a good idea to focus and stay focused until I have moved forward in my activity and how well I can do it. From time to time, I have bad thoughts about everything. I just remember that it is unhealthy to get into a nonpositive frame of mind and need to remember to draw on the spirit for strength.

Sometimes it is hardest to get started, however, this is the way I have turned my mind to the task at hand. I often tell myself to keep going just for one more minute and I will rest afterwards, so this makes me push for some extra. It has its highs and lows and I really want this to improve my situation, so I pray to be strong in character and endurance. I need patience because it takes time, and I am taking a long time, therefore, I won't give up and try not to think too much about how long it will take. Remember that Rome wasn't built in a day.

I have become dedicated to my health which is a by-product of my routine bedding in, and it only comes second to worshipping Jehovah. What I do is not perfect, and I am not stupid enough to think it is, but I know it has a chance and that is all I need to know. The chance is that it slows down any difficulties with my motor functions increasing. Sure, I am standing at the foot of a mountain, and I am intending to climb it. What does it matter if I don't reach the summit? It's not a race either but a marathon and I am doing my best. It is just I am personally up to getting as far as I can however huge the task is.

This is the attitude I stand by, and it can be hard to motivate myself but the longer I last, the better and easier to get started on this activity. It is okay to be late to start a routine and sometimes I am so tired because of the MS or medication or a combination of them both. It is okay to feel like it is hard work trying to maintain it too because it is a big task. If I give up, though, then I won't achieve anything, and with the amount of effort I have invested in it, I want to finish. It would be like starting a jigsaw and then halfway through putting it back in the box because you get bored with it. The only times I miss out on my workout is if I am ill or have a prior appointment so I could say I have a letter from Mum to miss it on some occasions. I can always squeeze it in if I have some spare time anyway. It is possible to find a solution to your problems my giving it some thought and appraising all the different approaches. So, think things through from start to finish and don't be prepared to accept something half-done.

Each day, I start with the perspective of my situation and what I need to do so that I can improve it. If I am hungry, I eat. If I am thirsty, I drink and if I am tired, I sleep, and it is the same for exercise. If I am unfit and get out of breath, I exercise. I need to add to these actions that I am ill with MS and must exercise, so if I haven't done it for the day yet, I should do it. Basically, having MS in my mind means I am always unfit and need to exercise. Being positive means believing things will get better and having the right state of mind. So, I keep to my routine and feel it is beneficial to me, so this is going to be how I get better at everything. I think I am being active and if I keep doing this, I will repair my functionality and I want it more than the time and effort I put in. It is the process of what the body is capable of and comes down to mind over matter. I have decided to fight MS and it is my responsibility to undertake what I can, so this is how I fix my mind on the topic. The body is remarkable and can overcome a lot if you put it to work and this is what matters, so you put it to work because you know it is the best option. All I need to do is persist in regular exercise and a healthy lifestyle, and it may start small, but believe me, it will grow. This is very good for the mind so nurture a belief that you can do it no matter what it takes. It is not merely the needs of the body such as food and drink, it is a state of mind and we can all gain a viewpoint that will make us act positively. Whether I enjoy it or not while doing it, I sure enjoy completing a session And feeling that the effort was worth it for the outcome. I have overcome doubt about the point of it all which can lead to even darker places and found a positive mindset. I must keep hold of this way of thinking and not fall down a rabbit hole of doubt. Building this into my life has taken time and patience and so I needed to push and push to reach the way of being happy with myself. I guess the danger lies in feeling happy with doing nothing. The reward is down to me and how far I am willing to go, and I can see the results as I go.

I have taught myself over time what to do with my health to improve it and I coach myself. It has taken tremendous amounts of belief and understanding of the consequences of doing nothing. I need to realise that I want to achieve results and that the time it will take to happen is yet unknown but I still carry on regardless. Everything is a learning opportunity And knowing that I am doing something actively to promote my well-being is very pleasing.

Perhaps there may come a time when new medication and treatment fixes me, but until then, I prefer to work in unison with the treatments and keep myself as active as possible. This gives me the reason to get up each day and follow a routine. I enjoy dreaming of a cure and I also get a rush from exercising which is always beneficial to your health.

From time to time, I must adjust everything I do and the thought of managing a routine stops it from getting boring but that will stay with me in one way or another. The longer I stick with the exercise routine, the easier it becomes to look after my health in that way. Although my limitations are not necessarily visible daily, if you compared me ten years ago to what I am like today, you would be able to see a distinct difference. All I want to achieve involves persistence and patience and I am proof of that for now. Keep this in mind and there is a reason behind maintaining a healthy routine. It feels like my treatment for MS and a good exercise routine are two different items. I have a routine and am happy to continue with it whatever my situation.

Meditation is a good way to relax and focus and keep on top of my life by treating the emotional effects of my condition. There are so many ways to meditate, and it is good to slow your body down, release tension properly in each part of your body and let your mind empty of thoughts and just ignore everything that comes to mind. I find it lowers stress and improves concentration and happiness and it is important to keep me from the depths of despair that can wash over me. I give time each day to muse over my life and muse on the happiness of prayer and peace. Some days, I spend an hour in the bath meditating on how things can be improved through the right medication, and this is food for blood pressure and circulation. The improvements I feel from meditation give me a great addition to my lifestyle and my body needs the rest. Remember to breathe steadily during meditation, even if you are using different breathing techniques involving changes in speed and intensity.

I also use different techniques of meditation and they fit into my life where needed and stop me from doing nothing useful when I relax. Whether I am looking to rest, work or play, I can get in the right frame of mind using various meditation techniques. So, I spend time each day being alone with my thoughts and focus on something in my life that perhaps is troubling me and that way, I can deal with it, so I feel better and am not letting it affect my conscience. There are ways to be sure that I am fighting the effects of MS with my behaviour and not just relying on medication to solve everything. The ultimate purpose is to have a mind that is healthy and therefore, has the correct outlook. It is important to recognise that I am using a combination of ways to deal with MS, and this importantly keeps my mind active and helps maintain peaceful and balanced thinking. There is a risk that an inactive mind can lead to boredom and depression especially when it is filled with some of the rubbish on TV. Try and be as occupied with a variety of activities as possible to be at peace. I don't spend too much time on one job or activity. As they say, "a change is as good as a rest".

If I can get outside and spend some time there, I find it very calming and I am thankful. The smell of grass and flowers helps to ground me and relax me and take me away from my body's aches and pains. Listening to wildlife like birds and bees is excellent too, for the same reason. It is a good idea to try and get outside at least three times each week to feel better. When in an environment of just nature, with no sound of traffic or people, I like to breathe deeply and listen to all the natural sounds, plus feeling the sun on my face and the breeze blowing against my skin is wonderful. I can feel angry thoughts leave my head and peace and happiness take their place. I admit that I do enjoy a storm with dark skies and lightning and the sound of rain beating on my windows, so I like all the different sounds of nature that are available. I find there is something therapeutic about all the noises and flashing lights of nature. Although it is often nice to look at snow in the winter, I will not go out in it because my balance is poor, and I will fall over without a doubt. I need to wear suitable footwear in the rain and assess whether it is safe, and the temperature is important due to heat dehydrating me and affecting my movement.

I think all this behaviour is helpful in maintaining a good perspective for times when life gets tough and it helps me remember the duties I need to maintain and why. Every opportunity to go out and experience things, or just watch, is vital. The activities can improve my outlook, and I know they will, over time, keep me at peace. However, I must not forget to consider the details of my situation and be controlled in what I do. Sometimes I forget to take things carefully and, in my mind, I allow myself to make the wrong decision because I think it will be okay. I must be smart because of my condition and need to remember to think about the risks and avoidances. I am past the time in my life when I act without considering my condition and am into a time when how I need to prepare for problems Is more important. MS is a problem I can't forget and I must accept that it needs consideration. I am always learning to live with these new changes and finding ways round them so that I can continue to enjoy life.

The diagnosis can hit hard and cause all manner of bad anxiety and stress, so, at the end of the day, remember to keep it real. Begin by learning everything you can and especially how you are affected so that you can learn to live with the condition, and you can survive. Don't waste time trying to work out a way to cope without including the treatment available. Make sure to deal with any physical and emotional problems you face before they escalate and, over time, see how you can work them in your favour like using changes in mood to stimulate meditation and prayer. It will take a lot of time for the most suitable medication to be selected and for you to get used to it and you can use this time to your benefit too by maybe researching the condition and exercising. Any ways to think positively are good, just don't focus completely on this – remember to add in some action too. Also, remember that your feelings will change over time and you need to take this into consideration when looking at what you are doing.

Like everything in life, if I spend too long thinking about what to do, I run the risk of doing nothing which is no help. It is all part of my life with MS, and everything has its use, from planning the time medication is taken to how long I am exercising. I don't want any regret or stress to manifest in my life when I have more pressing matters like remembering to take my medication, how much and how often. I identify the items which are causing ill feelings and resolve them or move on and discard them, so this way, I am happy and do not let myself dwell on bad thoughts. The mind must be taken seriously and treated well to be clear and confident. I benefit from a positive attitude and my environment is all a part of it, so I prioritise everything there is to prioritise. The more organization in my life, the less I worry. Think about how the brain and body are connected and how the right attitude can improve how the body feels and vice versa.

I have spent so much time thinking about the negative side of MS and understand it well. Whatever happens, enjoy your life, and have ways to achieve this, even simple ones like going out for a coffee. Try not to be coerced into doing things that make you worry. God knows how much time I have wasted thinking about my life being over and that was wrong, and I needed to snap out of it and start living the best I can. I can think of how I was able to do so much more and the sacrifices I have now made, and that the sacrifices have only really changed my ways. I could spend too much time thinking about how life would be different if I never suffered from MS, but what's the point? It is there and I need to address it. I like to think about how I am now so occupied with my body and mind's health and how much I have gained. I could look back at my life and imagine ways I could have done things differently, which is just something we all do. However, it is more important for me to figure out That there is plenty of time to find ways to deal with MS and plenty of things I can change too. I am letting the past go so that now I am free to try a new start and find a successful direction. I have spent time thinking and then planning and then making a move like I do when I play chess. I have decided to see what the future holds and not waste time on the past and instead, spend time focusing on my health and how to improve it. Basically, I live in the now and dedicate my effort to being able to give a routine I've worked on a chance to work. I think there are always possibilities if we look for them.

Now, prayer gives me the opportunity to offload all my troubles and leave them behind in the hands of our heavenly Father. It is as simple as leaving my problems with God to deal with for me and forgetting about them because I trust they are in good hands. Why do I care what people think about me or are saying behind my back when all I care about is our heavenly Father? The unseen things that God does are kept front and centre of my mind through prayer and not people. I feel the warmth of Jehovah's loving kindness, and this brings me tremendous strength in the knowledge that he is always available. The thing to remember is Jehovah is always there and, no matter the time, I can pray and get things off my chest. I make prayer a part of everyday activities, not that there needs to be a set time or place to pray. It doesn't matter when or where I pray, just that I pray. I am confident that I feel more positive in life thanks to prayer. I am at ease with my belief, and it gives me satisfaction that I am making time for daily prayer. In life, it can get hectic, and I can lose track of time easily with all my actions and forget to take medication, for example. The most satisfying things I do are pray and meditate because they give me calmness and help me to keep focused on what is important and not get distracted. When I was growing up, the times I wasted on pointless activities are countless and I have learned from that. Prayer is a good form of meditation and finding peace. It is a very good idea to learn to pray and by that, I mean think about what you want to pray about and just do it. When a person has a lifelong illness, they need to get busy living with it and all it involves, which can be overwhelming. So keep working on it and eventually, the problems the illness raises will become smaller and easier to handle.

I won't allow myself to be pulled all over the place trying to do everything at once when instead, I just focus on one thing at a time and that gives me the best ability to do a good job rather than stopping and starting something else multiple times. I make sure that I complete everything because I don't want to pick up half-done work later and realise what I was thinking about that distracted me from the work. I think it is important to not start work when there is not enough time to complete it and so I find something else to do instead until there is time. If I start something, I will finish it and do my best before I move on. It is important that I keep control of my life because an out-of-control life causes an unsettled and out-of-control mind. If I am trying to do everything at once, I am going to struggle anyway and this will cause stress and especially mistakes that never look good. Why am I trying to do everything at once anyway when I have the time to do things separately? Maybe I am in a rush so this is a good time to realise how to choose the most important items and just do some for now. Until I can do work, it may be necessary to just break the job into parts or get some help with it. I think and prioritise to the best of my ability, and this helps me avoid such problems because I want to maintain peace and satisfaction. Short of an emergency, I keep my head on my shoulders, and if I have too much to do I need to ask for help and not be so proud and think I can do everything myself and the right help is welcome.

The Bible teaches that there are problems inherent in people and we have the strength to be good and do what is right and keep calm or there are consequences. I never did this as a younger person but now I do what it takes with one objective and that is success and a good standard of life. Think like a winner and it will give you an attitude to win so you work hard to achieve this even if it doesn't happen straight away. Think like an algorithm and only guide the happy thoughts into your life and they will multiply. For so many years, I have just pushed myself over the edge and not thought of the consequences until it's too late. I have learned from my mistakes and with good guidance from people with experience. Do what is right and proper to be successful and remember not to overdo it and give in. Plan the jobs that need doing and, when there is time, move on to new jobs, but remember to complete the old jobs before starting new ones. Don't take on too much – remember there are others who can help to finish the job.

I have decided to move on and not remain stationary with things. I am not afraid of hard work, and I keep doing my best, not just for myself but for others. I take days as they come, and some are hard due to my routine. If I am with others and enjoying their company, I hope my determination will make others happy and positive too. Motivation is driving me to do more and more each day and I know I am improving. As I do more, the easier it becomes and the more volume I can handle. The more my attitude is to succeed and the more I find I am acting this way, the easier and happier I am. It is like practising a musical instrument and how it becomes easier and easier to play if you stick with it. I am sticking with a new life and that is important. I understand I need to keep my routine together and that is what counts so I don't think I will ever be able to stop without thinking about what the point was of starting in the first place. If I have doubts like this, I carry on anyway and I soon realise the magnitude of my work and how small everything else is. The basics are in place, and they will remain in place, and they will allow me to survive and give me the necessary time and direction to keep working on them. Every day, I am feeling more confident about keeping doing what is right in life. The basics are important, and they are my platform to grow from. It is time to get busy living. Without a desire and direction, I would struggle but fortunately, I find loads of positive emotions to draw on. When a job needs doing, and if you can provide the right attitude, there is no stopping you. Attitude can be a valuable tool for the task.

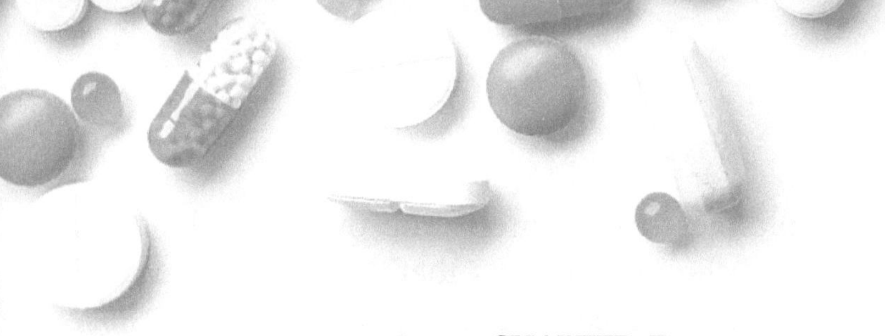

CHAPTER 7

Don't shut yourself away from people

Involve yourself in a society who are interested in you and encourages you and supports you because it makes an emotional difference in you. Don't think you can't get out and enjoy yourself because you can. It is worrying that even today, the attitude and treatment some people are subjected to and put up with are because of their health or age. If an opportunity to spend whatever time available with other people is there, it will be most helpful to get involved in it. Okay, things have changed for me but that doesn't stop me from a new life involving new things. I have found charity organizations that give me opportunities to take part in uplifting discussions. Attitude is changing, albeit slowly, and it is for the better so just be patient if alone and keep looking for opportunities. I've worked for many years with MS, and I always felt that the treatment I received changed from pre- to post-diagnosis and from okay to not okay respectively. I don't think much of the average employer as a result, however, it all happened under one employer and so I wouldn't tar them all with the same brush. From my experience, the average employer is more interested in money than welfare though and employees can treat each other cruelly when unchecked. Maybe they think they are helping to keep the business going or whatever and that is a fair point.

I try to let people meet me before I drop the truth about my health and that stops the assumptions that'll centre around MS like we are all the same and need a lot of help. I am aware of those employers who dismiss people due to disabilities and get away with it and this is probably because the employees don't know their rights and so it goes unreported. Generally, this is what people think and it is the most convenient way because it keeps things simple. I mean the way medical treatment is going, the chance of employing or just knowing a person recovering from disability is slim for now but getting more likely. So why doesn't society just accept them as they are? Are there people who see disabilities as a threat? What are the expectations of society? Generally, we are more accepting than we were hundreds of years ago though and are still changing for the better. I hate to say it but it seems to be older people who feel disabilities are a problem due to the education they had a long time before the advances in medicine. Basically, people stop and don't keep up to date with things as much as they could. This is probably caused by the media and ways to see just fragments of information being the way these days. There is a risk that people will only ever know bits of information. These are the people who don't care and maybe they are trying to be smart and are missing the mark. I think illnesses or disabilities are just part of life and shouldn't be a reason to avoid those suffering. Instead, we should be as involved as possible.

If I hear the words "because they have MS", or any other illness, it means discrimination to me. This is what you need to put up with when you are disabled so be strong-minded and try not to let it get to you. What do I care what a person thinks about MS anyway? The best thing for me is to be around people and to feel accepted. I want to work because it gives me meaning and financial help, which is welcome, I will put up with the opinions of others because I need to focus on what I am doing and know there are alternatives, and therefore if it is time to move on, I can. I can use the opportunity of employment to demonstrate that I can work. I don't want to feel that I depend on benefits; I want to be able to provide for myself, and there comes a time when you may need to push yourself to do this because of everyone around you. When you are constantly harassed by work colleagues about your abilities, and even ridiculed, it's okay to leave and live off benefits while finding someplace more suitable. I am not going to shut myself away because of them. I think from experience that I am going to have a real struggle but it is often the best choice not to give up. Therefore, it is down to me to fight for myself, and that way I know what is going on in the world of work.

In the past, I was guilty of thinking less of those in my situation and just fitting in with the crowd. However, I have the knowledge needed now to stand up for myself and I know when to quit which comes with age. I am trying to work with volunteer organisations to keep busy when I can because they are very understanding and thankful. The best advice is to stay calm and engage in the conversations as they happen and educate people who are misguided about disabilities. I am open and upfront about myself which makes me proud. I don't understand other people sometimes, so I just avoid them. I tell you this that I need to make some adjustments and I hope that is understandable. I have issues and there are things I am doing about them. Many people get to a point in their lives where they have an opportunity to support their family and need to understand they should give some kindness to others as well. The people who think entertainment and material possessions are more important than friendship are never going to be happy. We will all need help someday.

There is death and hurt and problems with health everywhere and they are often what people target and I feel that is out of fear. The best-case scenario is to talk and be with others and if there is a stage in life when this is not possible, don't get down but keep trying something new. This is a fact of life, and we are all the same no matter our age or wealth. Wake up and see this is the truth and the world we live in is broken. Don't live a sheltered life and only surround yourself with a certain type of person who is like you in their thinking and age - talk with everybody. If we all mix with different creeds and races and ages, everything would be beautiful. Imagine harmony and love among everyone. There would be no more war or poverty. I believe this will happen one day and there will be no wickedness anymore. Psalm 37, verses 8, 9: 'Just a little while longer, and the wicked will be no more; You will look at where they were, and they will not be there. But the meek will possess the earth, and they will find exquisite delight in the abundance of peace.' There is truth in this scripture and because Jehovah doesn't lie, we know it will happen. This will involve everybody so we can all work together on it instead of working on ourselves. I want to have people imagine themselves in my situation and then consider how they can help so they have empathy. I don't want people to imagine themselves in my position and then think that it is too much bother to help me and leave it to someone else. If everyone thought like that, then nobody would help others at all. A truly diverse society would include and not exclude people. We will look back one day at those who don't care and see how this was the problem with the world back then. It is important to see the error in not caring for others. If everyone wants somebody to do things for them, then we have a problem, and it will not help the changes that need to take place. Sometimes, someone needs to take the initiative and make the first move. Thank God for people who understand this and care enough to help whatever the cost. I will say that we all need to get on board before it's too late. If we don't care about others, we are going to end up in ruin as a people. We are meant to bring peace and reconciliation into our world.

My bad days may come across worse than they are, and I don't give up which must say something about me. I refuse to stop until I have no other option in my pursuit of the new me. When I was working, the company knew about my condition and what they think of me now since we have lost touch is of no interest to me. They should have focused on what I could do instead of what caused me issues. It is important to me to prove that MS means I can work because anything can be done and all it takes is effort.

There are ideas I need to use, and these are that I must find something I am comfortable with and that while I am looking, I can use my spare time to achieve something as well, like learning a language or maybe playing a musical instrument. I want to prove this to other people and myself and that even while out of work, I am being productive. We put men on the moon, so bear that in mind and understand that we are more than capable of dealing with difficulties and finding solutions to them. I have skills and knowledge I am keen to use and if people say I can't because of MS, then, in the words of Craig David, "I'm walking away". Working with MS is not impossible and can at most be a challenge and so find a job that supports you and helps find solutions by being positive and helpful. There are preferred jobs because they are less challenging for me and if my fellow workers are supportive and don't ridicule me, it will work out. I am willing to do most things and obviously, there are things I am more suited to. It would be beneficial to do work in which I have experience and need little training and just a bit of adjustment to get on with. How can I live a normal life with so much discrimination? I guess irresponsible employers are not interested in helping their employees and may reap what they sow. Has it come to that? I don't believe that there isn't an element of goodness in people. There are definitely some who go out of their way for others, otherwise, I would have given up long ago. Not having a job is not the end of the world, but it would be so good to *earn* a few beers at the end of the week like most people.

I am living as much of a normal life as possible without a job, and I don't think I am making a bad attempt at it. Overall, I am dealing with what is happening to me on benefits and if necessary, I can make cutbacks to my lifestyle and will find a way to do something to keep busy and cope emotionally. I am happy to think that what I am going through will yield positive results in some way that I can't quite see yet, but I am in it for the long haul And I haven't reached my last resort yet. Also, I am trying to show that I am doing pretty well with day-to-day activities under my own steam and using my head. I am using all my spare time to engage with society and feel normal again and getting out is key to this. Although in the past, having a job was key in my life, I now realise that I have many other options than just going to work for some company. If society at large provides the benefit to those of us working hard to fit in with others, then the world would be a better place because this is how most of us are even if we make some wrong decisions. I hope that it is noticeable to people who know my condition that I am doing well and that if they are interested in me and want to get to engage with me, they can. If life gives you lemons, then make lemonade. I am working hard, and I hope people see that and that it shows others that there are always options. I would like to think that I can inspire people with health problems like MS or diabetes to take the challenge and not give up hope, but instead, to do what is needed. This is a flag we can fly to show society we carry on and there is no reason to give up on ourselves. If anything, I hope to show by my own example that MS can have as small an impact on your life as possible, how I am dealing with it and who is there to help. Don't shut yourself off but consider doing things differently as there are people available to support everyone. A change in my course doesn't mean a change in the destination. I have made the necessary changes to help me carry on and I still want to arrive at the original place even if the journey has changed. This can be challenging, but everyone needs to be aware that although it seems complex, it doesn't need to be and they too can have an enjoyable and fulfilling life.

There is so much wrong with the way that people with disabilities are treated. It is hard to think that I am maybe never going to be treated normally again, so I don't think about it. I am positive, however, that things can turn out for the best and I can be happy that my routine is doing some good and that I can achieve new accomplishments by sticking with it. When I am dealing with people who know my condition, I only ask for or accept help when I need it. I think people are only trying to be nice, but they would help me if they let me ask for support and didn't just push it on me. I am trying to socialise with many people and feel I need to tell them about my health to allow them to understand my unique condition. This is personal for me and gives people the chance to learn that I am an individual with individual needs and not to be treated as part of a group. I just don't want to feel that I need to go around deceiving anyone about my health and feel I can be upfront and honest, so I can be looked on as me and not anything else. If the average person consistently treats me wrongly, then I will walk away, and they will never hear from me again, or at least for some time. If a person feels everyone with MS is the same, and that is what some people are happy to think, then don't let me stand in their way. I am sure I can find an organization out there that cares and understands what I am achieving and gives people respect for what they achieve and are happy to have them involved. I won't give up and roll over because that is what people think I need to do and because I have MS and hear about the problems this condition can cause. I am learning about the different opinions people have and often, these are due to their upbringing. I can't hold that against them but it's never too late for them to learn that they are mistaken. All I can do is my best and hope they see that I am unique, like everyone else, so I will try to be an example whenever possible. There is a chance that a person is told what they can and can't do so often that they start believing it or at least agree because it is easier. That is not good and even though it is hard work sometimes, I carry on flying the flag for equality. I am confident that people will value honesty and that I physically show my abilities. The important thing for me is that *I* decide when I need assistance and nobody else does. Sometimes, people just don't get that I am trying to live my life without help, So if I want or need assistance, I will ask for it – my choice.

Are we not all equal and it is just we may need to all be treated individually? We all have something to offer and there are organizations that will benefit if they embrace the fact that we are all the same with different experiences. I often wonder why society tends to label everyone into groups for convenience. Don't be narrow-minded like this and instead, enjoy the rich tapestry of life in all its splendour. Nobody but me knows how hard I am pushing to be on top of MS and there is no way it can be assessed by looking at other people, only me, and I will need to be studied a lot like everybody. I like to think my drive has shown how much I want to make a success of my current goals and I can encourage others to be the same with their ideas. This is the life coach in me. Sure, a person may think they know about me, and I want to meet that person and show them first-hand what I can do when I put my mind to it. This is another example of how eager I am to get out and meet people. They will notice the changes I have made in my life and accept them and see what is possible rather than assuming things from limited knowledge.

Some people smoke and drink and I accept this because it is their choice. I don't assume everyone who smokes is the same, and I know because I smoked for ten years and regret it but have beaten that. I'm worried that even though I quit in May 2002, I may have caused damage to my lungs which will affect me later in life. I have only myself to blame for my past and can now share advice on what I went through. I feel strongly that I should do things for myself, and other people should be aware that they are in control of their own destinies, depending on what they decide to do. So, a good understanding is important. We all make mistakes so why is it any different when I do? Apart from that, I have MS and that seems to be what some people focus on. I am saying to those who use MS as a reason to stop it if I trip because lots of people trip. I am being personal about things in my situation, and I hope most people don't have any problems with discrimination because it can lead to isolation and that is not healthy.

The sort of person that thinks life is all about getting drunk and having fun may be alarmed to know that society has viewed them as a separate section of society, and they are viewed differently from the average person. If I think about it, then different sections of society fit together better than others. Does my section fit with more sections than others? I hope my section fits with all others because I have optimism so we can enjoy each other's company when there is a chance to get together and do so.

It is likely that society hasn't met many a fighter like me and, therefore, they think the way they do about disabilities when they think of me, but I don't think I am a one-off. There are lots of people who are trying to become something even though they are in a difficult situation. I need to be one voice among many who prove that it is not impossible to do okay with difficulties and that we want to be involved as much as possible and not left out and alone. I am doing everything I can to set an example for all and inspire those who have given up caring about getting back into the game or staying a part of society. I am sure there are others who have a similar approach as me and want to socialise if they can and let people give them a chance. The main thing is not to get pushed aside for your differences and try to stay involved with others because it is so important. Whatever problems you suffer from, it would be nice to hear a well done from people and how inspiring you are to others whose needs are also something they need to work on, or even if you are simply inspiring to everyone. If mistakes are made, then what is wrong with a 'don't worry, give it another go' rather than 'you can't do that' which sounds like saying to someone that they can't get better. Find the time to think about what you can do and do it and don't let people judge you for you don't judge others and want to be like them. Sometimes, things would be better if people just encouraged you to help them and felt no pride in doing this. Pride is overrated and all thanks should go to our heavenly Father. There are very caring and supportive people around who understand it like this, and we should see that this is how everyone could be and not keep those who struggle at arm's length because they are a bad influence. We should be one big happy society where everyone is equal and, if some need extra help, it is available. I feel strongly that there is so much corruption in people who think only of possessions or of power and how they are only ever going to treat you with discrimination if you can't do things without help. Don't worry about this too much and instead, think about the society that will agree to let you be a part of its community, warts and all. I keep looking and seeing this around so don't think poorly about yourself.

Those who don't care much for disabled people are something of a challenge as far as changing their opinion. If you are one such person, then wake up and smell the coffee because you may find you develop some illness that is life-changing and an opportunity to learn from people with one such condition has passed you by. We should live together in harmony because the future can change big time and I am an example of this. It is quite a sobering thought, and I am talking from experience because I would say I was without any real problems for over thirty years and lived a selfish life. As a person who has been through what I have, if I know a person with a serious condition, I want to see how they are coping and how they are supported. They are then influencing me, and I am going to want to spend time around them to learn and I want to ensure that nobody who knows me feels alone. Even if it is only a phone call, if I do this, It shows that I am keeping myself involved, and not giving up on myself or others. In the way that I find spare time for exercise, I will find spare time to talk with people. As I keep saying, it is time for action and to show what I can do and see what others can do and that is why I am keeping busy and engaged with people. I want to inspire those who need to do something and, like me, have time on their hands and can be there for each other and therefore not alone in life. Look, my life is not over; it has just changed me and that will happen to anyone as they age anyway so take note. If there is at least some unity out there in the world, I will keep going out and socializing over coffee and/or cake. Let's face it, I'm trying, and I hope that is infectious. So, I am not happy if I am not part of a community and there is nobody to talk to even if just for a minute.

Education about MS is available to everyone so if you know someone who has the condition, don't waste time on pity – learn about it and show empathy instead. I can spend half an hour a day learning anything I like and, all the while, there are people wasting their time getting drunk and misbehaving as if it is a better use of time. We are living in the age of the internet and a person could spend half an hour learning about MS to support someone they know with MS rather than looking at entertainment or possessions they want, for example. I'm sure anyone could make the effort for half an hour a day.

Even in a company, if they employed someone with a condition like mine, surely the Human Resources department would find out about it from professionals, not from friends. I mean if you needed an operation, you would want a surgeon to do it, right, and not your friend? I hope lots of people with deaf children would learn sign language, or are there people who wouldn't do such a loving thing? Although there are parents who neglect their children, and thankfully there are agencies to deal with that, this is rare. Well, I think we all have an obligation to each other. A responsible employer would keep up to date with the needs of their employees and show an interest in one who has health issues when they're at work. If they didn't, I would consider them to be unqualified and wonder how they got their position. I would hate to think that this person only thinks about their employees negatively to see how they can gain more out of them so they can increase their profits. I guess it's true that with power comes corruption and I want this to change and instead be responsible and show in their mission statement. Well done to people who spend their lives amassing money and then die and have spent no valuable time with their family and friends. Talk about missing the point!

From my position, I am interested in the lives of people who are suffering from lifelong conditions because I want to involve everyone and am willing to do anything I can to support them. I like to see the way they are coping with life and are not giving up on being a part of society. That is one thing they don't need. Many people go through life-altering situations and can still contribute to society. It may never be the same for them due to responsibilities in their won circumstances, but they have learned how to live with it. They have taken the advice to be able to know a safe way to continue in their life, and importantly, they know when to have a break and rest and regain what independence they can. It is important to talk to medical professionals about any limitations you may need help to overcome, and the health professional will get you support if it is needed. I have come across plenty of people who, without actually knowing me, tell me what to do or what I need instead of offering an opinion. Medical professionals are going to assess each case and make professional decisions so all they need is your input and they never treat you as anything other than an individual. If people need help to understand how to deal with a challenge, then they must get help and not just imagine what to do. Look past the walking stick or size of print they read and see the person and that is important for us all. If you get off on telling people information without any research involving that person, then you are a fool, and therefore, more than just this person's opinion is necessary. I know society may focus on the time and monetary cost this may incur, and this is limiting the field of workers that are more than willing to work hard at overcoming obstacles and is losing out. The people being overlooked have experience and knowledge and are so unique that they are worth the difference they make and the encouragement they bring. Many people don't think twice about taking time off work for a headache and I don't think that way about MS causing a loss of work so what does that say? Possibly material possessions have become more important than we think and that is a shame because being around people is priceless. It has taken my illness to work this out and some people never work it out. Look, I can show people these answers and I don't make them go through the same trials as me. Can people show me the time?

There is a definite problem with people in some parts of the world not wanting to look after each other as if it is easier to let someone else do it. This is the challenge and I only hope that one day, someone like me doesn't run the risk of being isolated. For example, I was made redundant when my employer could have left me on furlough for a year. It was available to them and would not have cost them a penny. I couldn't understand how they could justify that – even a ten-year-old could have worked that one out. Maybe they panicked or were given poor advice, and, in all honesty, I am long past caring. If they had so much to deal with and it was a time issue, then they could have delegated the work. However, I knew them well and the only reason they had their position was because they were born or married into the owner's family. Also, I think sometimes that my own father would cut me out of his will and leave everything to my only brother and if that happens, it is a sign that he didn't love me back. The thing is, we used to talk to each other a lot and he would always say he was going to make a will and leave everything to me and my brother and that he needed me to sign it. However, since then, this conversation topic just stopped ever occurring and that's when I started thinking that he had already made this decision. Even my sister-in-law's parents left something to their grandkids. Is this an example of money being more important than life? I could be just enjoying a bit of speculation though. Am I just becoming paranoid? If he had never mentioned it, I would never have let it cross my mind.

Is ours a society that does not want to care for disabled people and instead wants them cared for by other people? Don't marginalize people; instead, take an interest in their lives and who they are and what they can achieve. Look for the things about them that make them unique and show an interest because they are so special. Think about how precious a person is and realise they are priceless in life. Be willing to join them for a coffee and a bite to eat occasionally and go on your binges with your other friends before it's too late. Some people just don't seem to know how to get involved, thinking it is better not to, and of course there are those who take no notice of what you're going through. So the best line of defence is to be nice to everyone and keep involved with people as much as you can.

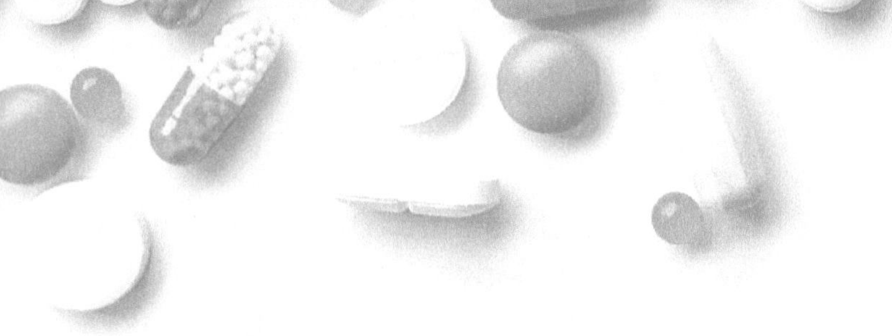

CHAPTER 8

Enjoy what you are doing

Concentrate on using the mind to keep seeing a job through and give it your best shot and this will create enjoyment. Find a way to think that is in line with your goals and this will keep you happy because the goal is going to be reached in some way. I have the attitude I need to make myself do what is needed and I believe it is possible to overcome my disability and that people can at least try to feel better, even if they don't try anything else.

The body is capable of great things, so if I can strive for improvement, then I am on the right course. Instead of using the word can't, use the word can and that helps to at least start thinking and trying to do your best. My attitude is positive, and I use it to help me put the extra work in and not give up and instead, leave it to other people to encourage me which is sometimes negative. When there may be nobody available, I will train on my own and this is where it is down to me for motivation and so it is important to do everything as normal myself. I can't expect someone to motivate me as much as I motivate myself. The way to train is always going to change as you improve your strength and stamina, and therefore, the activity will need changing to compensate. I have changed because my health changed, so I now fit things together and I will change again if it is needed because I know how. This is what it takes to keep me mentally limbered. I have taken note of what is involved in this sort of process, and this may be of use to me in the future. Due to making the necessary changes to my way of thinking, I know I can put in one hundred percent, and this makes me happy. I am being as fluid as possible to get through with MS and it is important to understand I don't always feel good until I get started, so getting started is necessary. I spend time where it is difficult, and thankfully, I don't require anyone to push me into doing what I need to because it is so odd not to do this myself now. If I don't put in the effort, I will not feel this way. I don't just do what I feel like and that is because I must mix things up sometimes and do what I need to do to accommodate when things change in my health. I see the benefit in what I am doing and looking for this is important if I am to believe in my success and feel happy with what I continue to do. When I feel I am improving in strength and stamina bit by bit, I can contemplate that it all adds up over time and all the bits make a big difference eventually. I am positive that over time, other things that I haven't even thought of will improve and that will be a joyful bonus. So, there is a belief that there will come more joy.

There are lots of people who will help me but I like to let them know that if it's an inconvenient time, I can try by myself first. However, this sometimes ends in trouble so it's important not to rush things. The Bible tells us of the Good Samaritan in the gospel of Luke which illustrates the care of a stranger. I see it on the news where people can be selfless and emotionally feel for others and are helping others and that is what I count on sometimes to support my activities. So, I am not worried too much about what I do which can be a hindrance. I have friends I can call on if I'm stuck and I know they will help when they can, but failing that, I also have support from medical professionals. I am pleased to take the help when I need it, but sometimes, when I think about things, I can work out the solution myself. Maybe I just dislike authority and that is partly why I don't listen to everything but it's important to show humility and not to be judgemental because I have been helped home a few times by strangers after running into difficulties. In the account of the Good Samaritan, we see how some people who have every reason to avoid each other are in a situation where one helps the other because they feel pity for them. So, sometimes you need to put your differences aside and get along with people because they are your best hope. Health and well-being are more important than what you believe and how you feel about people so try to stay friendly with everyone and you will have support there when you need it. In life, I have learned to prioritise and deal with situations accordingly and try to put everything in order of importance and this can be filled with joy if many others are involved. If I have a dislike for authority, then I need to deal with the root of that problem and not just leave it to fester. I should treat everyone equally and fairly and change the way I used to feel. The way to feel happy is to strive to treat others in the way you would like to be treated.

If you can maintain a positive outlook and are not afraid to try something new, then you won't regret not trying things or missing out altogether. Dealing with a health problem is tough and I am up for it both because it is good for me and will inspire others to try, no matter their issue. I will keep working in whatever form it takes and this will give me happiness because regret won't exist. It may feel like I am wasting my time if there are disappointments and maybe I should put things in a different order of priority. However, the key is to spend my time well and not waste it. For example, I can find the most beneficial use of time and that may not seem to be the most important, but I am trying and learning from it all. Spending time going to Bible meetings may not seem important to everyone, but it is giving me the hope and belief that I need so I will not go without it. Using my time effectively and keeping busy is best if I am aiming to be kept happy. So, I do rest because it is important, and I do spend time preciously. I am feeling the benefits.

My goal is to be in great health, all things considered, and this is going to make me happy because I will feel at my best. I feel much better when I am in good health and that is giving me plenty of motivation. The opportunity is available to me, and I understand what is involved so I am taking it by the horns and running with it. Basically, I am not squandering the time I have while off work. For my part, I start with my mind set on what I am trying to achieve and what that involves. Making the wrong choices will hurt and if it happens, I just remember it is not the end of the world and learn from it then carry on and adjust where necessary. I am living with a mind to optimise everything, but mistakes are part of learning and should be used in that way too. I take my time with what I do and how I go about in life because of my health, yet I will not let MS stop me completely. Keeping my brain free of stress and anxiety will be needed if I want to have a good attitude and so I keep occupied and don't let myself sit around doing anything unconstructive for this could turn into a habit. I need to focus on everything I do to make sure I do it to the best of my ability and am confident and it may involve changing what I am doing for a bit of time. Surprisingly, things do become easier if they are reasonably and regularly done and I don't give up any more thinking there is something better to do. I am falling into a routine in which my focus is firmly based on reaching my objective no matter how long it takes. This is a routine that has, over time, become part of my life.

Knowing what I am doing and why is important when keeping

focused and I get people who understand this is what is involved. When a person understands the reason I am doing what I do, it shows they have thought about it. I will fare better whatever happens if I don't panic because I don't want to lose control of my routine, so I think carefully about what I am doing and the order I do things from sunrise to sunset. There is no need to rush, and if a job is going to be done well, then take the time and enjoy the process. I didn't always have a goal, and it has taken time to get it to this place where it has become very important to me to understand that it is a marathon and not a race and I must keep going. Hold on to this and build on it because it is a foundation that will hold everything together. Things generally don't happen overnight, so patience is needed. For example, it takes time for me to get used to the side effects of new medications when I need to change them, and it is important to stick with them for a time and see how things eventually start working out. Don't forget, the body will become more tolerant in time and therefore, the way it started making you feel in the beginning will not continue. This is the same with exercise and it becomes easier to maintain the more you keep it up too.

I think of my situation as an opportunity and want to find what I can do with it and what it will do with me. I have spent lots of time thinking and that is good to get things straight and stops me from rushing into anything unprepared. At some point, though, it is important to start acting on ideas otherwise you can spend too much time thinking which will run the risk of becoming procrastination. Once you have thought things over, come up with a plan and go for it. I can't just put all my ideas to one side and there will always be some element of thinking throughout any action, but the only way I can achieve anything is with action and so I put everything into practice and take it from there. The way I think has now got a purpose and uses my drive and sense of purpose to progress. I want it to be a success and will stop at nothing to achieve this so I can meditate on that when I have a chance to help me keep going and not quit. This way to think will leave little room for negative thinking which is where all the cannots and doubts come from. Basically, I have given myself enough to keep occupied and not get bored. If I get bored, I inevitably stand a chance of doing something pointless so because I want to enjoy myself, I can use the time to practice a new skill like drawing and that is something I can come back to and do more of every time I feel bored. The idea is important to keep me satisfied and stop me from wasting valuable time doing nothing. I do get tired, and it is natural to have bad thoughts, so I always look to pray for strength and peace to help me get through times like these. If I get stuck with everything going on in my routine, I know I can pray for strength and peace wherever or whenever, so I can always find time to pray. The main goal is to start a routine and maintain it and be satisfied, and dedication will be invaluable for this. So build up your stamina and strength and you will enjoy how this makes you feel.

So, given what I am facing, I spend time thinking about how to act and then I use my ideas to find activities to try and work towards my goal of improving my health. Knowing that I am making good choices based on researching and developing an idea is important and needs careful consideration. I don't just act either without any thought because that is a recipe for disaster. It is important not to rush and try to do too much for this is how mistakes happen and time is wasted. A little extra time spent wisely goes a long way. Any ideas need to be thought about and then the appropriate action taken so make sure you don't get overzealous. Sure, it is reasonable to reflect on how things are going and that will enable a person to correct anything as needed. If I can keep this going, there may be some success and so I am optimistic about the outcome, and this is a discipline I use to maintain myself both physically and emotionally. Optimism is the key to achieving what I want in life and it works for most things, including my health. Think of what you can do instead of watching too much TV and how much you can achieve in half an hour and then spend half an hour less watching TV and try and achieve that something in the time.

It can be as simple as learning a new skill in that time or creating something and it is important to be honest with yourself. If a person lies to themselves, then things are going to go wrong in their lives, no matter what they do, so be true to yourself and everything will be so much easier. If I lie to myself about how much beer I drink, for example, then I will risk damaging my liver in the long term and making my health worse which will not bring me joy. I am just focusing on my health problem and giving it a chance at being controlled. This can't be a waste of time for anyone whether they are dealing with health issues or not. The act of making a change to take hold of an opportunity is a way to increase the control of an opportunity as it becomes available. Take hold of opportunities or they will turn into regrets. Be aware of opportunities and the right way to treat them.

Thinking and action are good exercises for my mind and body so even if I am not feeling good, I strive to get started and soon start to feel good again. I enjoy exercising my brain as well as my body and it makes me satisfied because I am not just benefiting my health but also my attitude and it makes me feel happy. Maintaining a good connection between body and mind can also be beneficial for functions such as coordination. For MS, improving coordination can be vitally important for giving back control to the brain, so try to limit pastimes that do not enhance brain power.

I always make sure I am in a healthy environment so that I am not putting myself at risk of being influenced otherwise. That can also help me to think positively, which, as I have already explained, can be so important in looking after your welfare. If I want the right attitude, I need to nurture this whole way I live so I am working on it and this is a positive thing to do. This means I am thinking about my health and giving it priority. Therefore, keep ensuring that a framework is in place that is driven by important things like healthy living and thinking and this will filter down to a happy life. Ensure the people around you know this and will not expect you to undertake unhealthy activities because they will be disappointed. Instead, focus on the people who support what you are doing and will not harass you into being unhealthy and know the reasons you make your choices and allow you to do so. What kind of person will tell you to do what they want if it is going to be detrimental to you? there are people who will want the best for you and will not stop you from doing things that are healthy and good for you. However, there are others who just want you to do what *they* want, so make sure you know where to draw the line. A person should respect and support you or leave you alone and spend their time with people who want to do a similar thing as them. Why would anyone not care about others being happy?

Be strong and stick to your decisions to try and beat MS through all that is happening, even when you feel you are losing the fight or missing out on entertainment. So far, I feel a whole lot better because I have started being more positive and I want people to see that I smile and enjoy what I am doing even when it is a struggle, and I will say that God willing, those events are working in my favour by giving me more drive. Maybe I can influence others who see how I benefit from my activities, and they will try to follow a routine of health and fitness set up in their schedule. It is important that I prioritise and realise the importance of some things over others. I hope that the message I convey is that I do this always and only stop temporarily and for a very good reason. After making a commitment to follow a routine, I make the effort to do so otherwise the process is not complete. It would be futile to go through the process of putting together a good routine if I don't start it and just put it on the shelf. Even if I make mistakes, it doesn't mean it hasn't worked – I just need to try harder next time or amend the routine to avoid any further errors. That is how it works with dedication to a purpose. Learning what works is a healthy way to use your mind and feel more involved mentally and therefore is part of the ongoing life of transformation. I am doing my best to make a new life and find an enjoyable one at that. Don't give up and think anything is impossible. Instead, stretch yourself to achieve goals above and beyond your activities and never think that you are doing enough and get comfortable. As a task goes, there are going to be lots of things happening and it is important not to lose the plot, and so, over time, and with patience, everything settles down. Sometimes, like many other people, I want to just lay around and do nothing, but I talk myself out of that and into my normal routine. Then, even if I don't realise it until I am finished, I get the positive vibe that I have achieved something and know that the effort has been worth it. A positive attitude is what you need to maintain, and dedication is what it takes.

I give myself targets to reach, or at least try to reach, and that keeps me going because I don't want to feel comfortable and get complacent when I should be trying to reach for more. Feeling comfortable is a way of losing drive and purpose so avoid this and instead, always work to reach new heights when you can. I get the most joy if I reach a target. Being positive is all in the mind so if I believe I can do a thing, I will keep trying to do that thing and hopefully achieve it and then set a new target. It would be remiss of me to think that I don't need to do anything to improve my situation because I just know I must. Is it possible to prove what I am doing is not helping without stopping and seeing what happens? I like to play chess, so I do that against other people online and am always trying to improve my game. This activity gives me patience and a drive to get better and, in many ways, this is like my life. In chess, I need to think a few moves in advance and there is a benefit to being able to do this and working out the result of making a few moves in advance helps so much. I don't let playing chess take over my life and just spend a bit of spare time each day, but I do it regularly and bit by bit, I am improving. When I am playing chess, it Helps with considering the options before making a move, a play which can be very useful in real life. It also teaches the benefit of forward planning and using time wisely. You see, life requires a sensible approach and then a sensible action and there is time available to be sure this is the best action. It is important to be satisfied with your actions and feel happy that they will benefit the future so understanding this is useful.

I do my best at everything and make myself happy with the process by seeing how it can benefit me and perhaps others in some way. The opportunity is available to me because I have the time for now and the drive to do what I can with the time. I still make mistakes and think this will always happen, so I don't let it get me down but instead, try and keep learning so that I do better in the future. Even for the things I struggle with, I am happy to add them to my list of things to do and monitor for improvement as part of my program. I don't want to omit things because I am not easily coping with them. Hopefully, I can become better and stronger and the times I struggle with certain activities will become a thing of the past. Now, looking over things I have achieved is much more rewarding, especially when I realise that parts of my routine have now become easier too.

After a night's sleep, I am at my best physically and will do what I can till I must rest again, and then I change from physical to mental exercising. The afternoon has become my best time to rest and a time for prayer and meditation. Enjoyment in how much I can do is a drug for me, and I am addicted and won't stop. There may come a time when I am going backwards in my abilities and that time will not stop me but give me a reason to make changes so that I can continue as best I can.

I get such a boost when I am improving in activities and actions, and even if I am struggling with parts of my routine, I look on the struggles as a way to prove to myself that I can get there if I strive to. No matter how small the advancement, I will put in the effort and be thankful – thankful that I am able.

It now feels as if I have been following this path for long enough now that I am set on it being my way to success. Therefore, I am happy that I am doing what I have conditioned myself to do to succeed.

Basically, I am convinced that I must continue because stopping is a bad idea. Enjoyment comes from the belief that I am doing everything in my power to have the best time and my health is a priority in this. I now do so much variety in my routine and it takes up so much of my time that I am confident I can overcome whatever obstacles life throws my way. It just goes to show that there is no need to give up because even if the way forward is hidden, it is there and you can find it. Enjoy the process of discovering and putting together a solution to anything that comes your way. The time will come when you see that what you are doing is enjoyable and you put all your doubts behind you. Think and calculate what needs to be done and this is an enjoyable process. There is enjoyment in life and what you do, so don't give up. Everyone will see this in you.

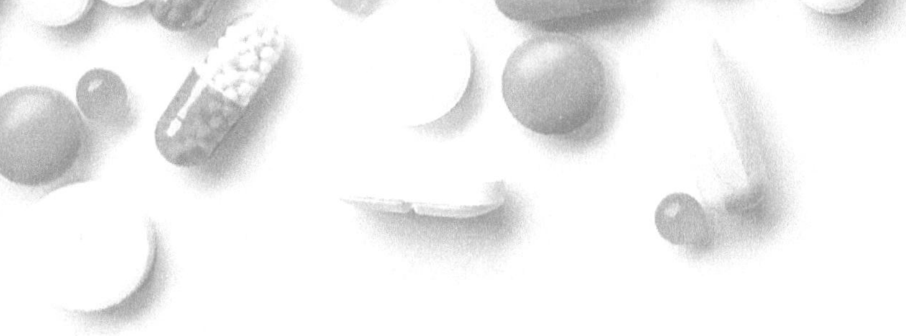

CHAPTER 9

Achieve a rewarding lifestyle

Being told I had multiple sclerosis took the wind out of my sails, as you can imagine. It was such a shock and a huge deal to me because I knew it was a life-changing illness. I thought it all through and realised it needed a plan of action focusing on making a success of what was left available in my new life. MS is an illness I didn't have much understanding of and so I thought it was game over at first. I didn't start planning my funeral or anything like that, but it was more like my useful life was over, and I thought I had been through my best years and all I could ever achieve, and that was as good as it would get for me from then on. It took time to come to terms with this news and, lucky for me, it isn't an aggressive type that I have, and I was properly able to start a routine of healthy living including a healthy diet and exercise. I needed time and preparation to move forward, and I spent what time I needed starting on medication and making plans I thought would help. Healthy living was the first move because the news made me start to think about how I wasn't leading the healthiest life and I wanted to give myself the best chances.

First of all, there was a lot of thinking about myself and what could work for me. One of the best things I decided was to never nap in bed. Once I am up, I stay up until bedtime at night. I might need to nap in a chair after taking medication, but the bed is for night-time.

Over many years, I have settled into a treatment routine that works best for me and has involved a lot of effort thanks to exercising and diet etcetera. When I was first told of the diagnosis, I didn't tell anyone for a couple of weeks and just found myself living in shock, so I needed to snap out of that and get on with life. Everything suddenly got intense very fast, and I wasn't totally ready, but would I ever be? This was life-changing news and gave me a feeling of mortality in a more intense way than ever before. There have been times I had feared for my life but nothing like this.

The MS team started me on disease-modifying therapy, and I began a new outlook on my life and wanted to do something to support this exercise as well as taking the medication. Obviously, it was early days, and only over time would the MS show itself in various ways, so I kept going to work each day like normal and only told a few people I worked with. this was fine but eventually, everyone had heard through the grapevine. I felt down for ages and think that is normal and so I needed to deal with that before moving on and prayer helped me with living with this feeling. Well, it took time, and I may never feel like I did pre-diagnosis again, but I kept on as normal because I didn't see any reason to change straight away without finding out more about how my life would be affected.

Initially, I was okay health-wise except for my left eye and this continued for the first few years. Things were changing slowly though, and I needed to come to terms with it, so I didn't want to add to my troubles with a poor lifestyle. I think the gravity of the change needed time to sink in and so I gave it time. I expect there are changes for us all over time and they will be big or slight, and fast or slow, so we are all similar in that respect. I wasn't prepared for this change in my life but thankfully, I was given time to work and am thankful that my situation wasn't impossible to maintain. Maybe I was naive and thought this would have happened to someone else, but in a way, I was fortunate that the change came quite slowly so I had time to amend my outlook I spent a lot of time trying to work out if I had done something to cause the MS, and Although I now know that there is no known cause, I still had to work through that for myself and have finally put that idea to rest.

Basically, MS would change my life completely but a bit at a time and the best thing I did was keep going through it all, even the hard stuff. It was not like a headache that would pass in a day or two with painkillers, unfortunately. The troubling thing is MS is big, 'rest-of-life' stuff, and it needs managing in a big, 'rest-of-life' way and involves learning how to adapt to change because this is important if I want to get it under control. I needed to start by getting used to this fact or I was running the risk of getting stuck thinking about how much my life had changed and potentially might continue to change. I really needed some emotional help to keep sane and this was available from the medical team who were wonderful and explained to me what effect it may have but how to focus on the now.

Over time, I could formulate a strategy, and this was going to take lots of time and when it's my health, I was going to give it lots of time. This was a coping mechanism where instead of admitting defeat and stopping living, I was going to live a healthier life. In the beginning, it was a bit hit-and-miss as I found my feet and what suited me best. I am working on breaking MS and have the rest of my life to work on it so no rush there. Lots of things went through my mind and were not all good and this is understandable but needs controlling. The best thing I did was keep myself busy and control my conduct. It is not a race, but I understand the need for medical and spiritual help to fit together with my work, and this is something that is best begun as soon as possible.

When I have time, I have a duty to put my lifestyle under the spotlight and this, as it turned out, is a brilliant thing to do irrespective of MS because more than anything, I can see what it lacks. I regularly consider my lifestyle now and adjust it when needed. These days, I am constantly thinking about exercise and diet because everything else was being taken care of already by my medical team. It is not too difficult to take a tablet each day. Exercise has benefits whatever your reason for it and it releases chemicals in your body that relieve pain and make you feel happy so is very beneficial to do. Hydration is key for life! Whether I drink tea, coffee, juice, or water, it doesn't matter; the idea is to take on board at least a litre of fluid each day. I now understand that whether I am thirsty or not, I need to drink fluids regularly during the day and make sure I have breaks to accommodate this. Don't worry too much about what is right and what works best because that is a learning curve that we need to stay with and find answers to. As time goes by, I Have found the best route for me to follow, and although this has taken years, I can't see it changing now. What is important is to stick at it and remember, there is a way for things to fit together that will suit anyone. Remember the reason you have decided to make these changes and that will become what you are trying to achieve, and the rest is down to you putting in the effort. So, keep doing what you can to slow down the problems you are dealing with and improve your health. The task at hand is going to hopefully become a daily habit instead of a task.

A healthy diet is very important as the last thing I want is extra illness heaped on top of MS caused by eating junk foods because that would add another dimension to my already complex problems. I enjoy a healthy amount of fruit and vegetables in most meals to make them as balanced as possible nowadays. Some days I abstain from meat altogether and just eat lots of things like potatoes and carrots which are so filling, and don't forget the bread because there is such a variety available. Of course, a person will feel depressed at times in their life, and they may just be tired or worried, so keep your mind busy and don't forget fluids and rest which all helps.

Being told you have something like MS is one upsetting event but you can find happiness with clean living because it impacts feelings due to the health implications. If I found myself stuck in a depression with no way out, it would be very bad, so I am convinced that I can get through it. Clean living is a good defence against depression because it keeps a person occupied with choices and is not harmful to the brain like too much processed food is. At times like these, it is very easy to look for a quick solution like an alcoholic drink or worse, so over time, learn ways to avoid these vices like using prayer and meditation and instead, keep yourself away from these temptations. Understand that this is the best course of action and is not necessarily the easiest and quickest and so do try your best.

Firstly, ask yourself what you want to achieve and have an objective in mind. "I want to beat MS and keep it in remission and am getting strength and confidence by meditating on trying and reaching this goal." I am only human, so I am going to make mistakes, and it's okay when this happens so don't fall into the trap of giving up on one error. On an occasion, I am partial to a burger with all the extras like fries and a milkshake and that doesn't happen much because I won't allow it to become a regular thing. I have spent enough time looking into MS and formulating a plan of action not to let it get away from me. I look for anything to do to keep me from boredom because this is where I will risk tripping up. I order good food in my home delivery to avoid having anything unhealthy near me should my resolve weaken. The only way I am going to eat rubbish is if I go out and it's okay if I treat myself occasionally because it gives me a chance to socialise and enjoy myself. The important thing is not to get carried away, and that is down to me so I must keep mindful of my goal. At home, I can always find something like cleaning and tidying to do. I am partial to reading and music so I can always entertain myself and avoid boredom. Perhaps I will put some music on when cleaning or washing and it all becomes more enjoyable and less of a burden. If the weather is nice, I can read outside and enjoy the fresh air. So, I am just using my head to find things to do and not get bored to the point of making mistakes with my health. There is always spare time, so I am not worried or stressed that I will run out.

Meditate and pray for understanding and support to help maintain a calm mind and a clear perspective and to keep everything in context. Do not rush the new lifestyle process but begin by speaking with friends and family for support in coping with MS to the extent that you may need without having everything done for you – you need to take an active part in looking after you!

Now, the decisions you make, like me, are normally long-term and especially when dealing with a long-term health condition and so they take time and must be done properly. I made choices and intended to stick with them and generally keep them even if I need to adjust some of my life to allow them to fit in. In the beginning, it can be difficult adjusting everything to fit, but over time, even if it keeps changing to a degree, you will find that you work out how everything fits within your plan. It is only natural to keep adjusting an action plan as things develop over time. Sure, I have lots to keep on top of so can start by writing down what the main activities are considering commitments like employment, and it may be a good idea to put a simple table like this together, which is what I use and includes the basic commitments and framework:

TABLE OF REGULAR ACTIVITIES

TIME	ACTIVITY
7 am	Wake up, have breakfast with fluids and take any medication
9 am	Work on the tower or equipment to help strengthen and take fluids
11 am	Make sure you are hydrated and feel okay so maybe rest a bit
1 pm	Eat lunch with fluids and take medication if required
2 pm	Further exercise to build stamina and take fluids and rest
4 pm	Chores and home maintenance to keep a clean environment
6 pm onwards	Eat supper and relax in spare time using meditation and prayer

The idea is to set up a tool that can be used and consulted whenever necessary to help you plan your days to get the best from them. I can add or change parts of this table where I want. Always feel free to add or change it to suit your circumstances due to your times and activities. It doesn't need to be a work of art because it is not for that reason - it just needs to give you an idea of the basic elements of the day and supply something to work around and help to frame the day with. This idea helps me to return to my routine if, for some reason, I have stopped for a while and need a guide to follow to get back on plan. This plan is not set in stone but can be used as a guideline for maintaining activities since we could all do with a reminder from time to time, however, it can be flexible enough to accommodate certain commitments such as medical appointments, etc.

Considering my diet, I think it is an important part of life and it is incumbent on me to maintain a healthy gut. I want to be healthy and so watching what I eat and drink can be a great way to stay on track as far as healthy eating is concerned. I am not perfect but if I can stay close to a healthy diet, I am okay. Eventually, everything comes down to making healthier choices rather than rushing to eat whatever is there, so it is worth thinking about when you are shopping. When I grew up it was down to my parents to encourage me to eat well, and I was at their mercy since they bought the food and prepared it, but thankfully, my mother did a pretty good job. The only problem was my father was easily coerced into buying junk and giving it to me and my brother. When I was a teenager though, I gained some nasty habits from friends that were not good for me and found that I ate from fast food places and had no regard for how much sugar or salt the food contained. I smoked, drank, and ate rubbish with impunity. I would not do this now as I have seen what is wrong with it because now, I feel a whole lot better about my diet. Eventually, over a long time I changed, and I was trying to eat and maintain a healthy life long before my diagnosis. I cannot suggest that MS has done me a favour and opened my eyes to a good diet or that MS was caused by it either. I am saying that a good and balanced diet is sensible, and I feel the benefits in how my body functions and it is lasting so I am glad. All I can say is that I am more eager to ensure my diet is healthy because I have MS. Who knows when or how long it took for MS to be apparent in me? If investigated, there are plenty of programs and books that will advise a clean diet and even though it is your choice, eating and drinking better can help you in the long run. I like to think that as I got older, I started to care about what I was eating anyway, and I gained an interest in healthy living for no other reason than it was a sensible thing to take up. As it turns out, I love fruit and eat lots of berries and nuts and my diet is brought about by trying different foods. After all, there is so much good food that grows from the ground to support life. My diet is rich in vitamins and minerals which are beneficial to us all so we can eat well from the bounty available. I have broadened my taste and I try new things and eat a varied diet strongly based on health. I have not tried everything that is available yet, but I can eat plenty of foods that I like from the ones I have tried. I still have plenty of time to try all the others which may be healthy for me. Also, it is a fact that my tastes have changed with age and perhaps I should listen more to what my body tells me. I am sure I like savoury foods more the older I get and am not such a fan of sweet tastes anymore; given the choice, I know what I would choose. I investigate eating fresh and nutritious food because I enjoy it and its health benefits are a bonus.

Exercise is an important part of my health and I think it is a part of my effort in surviving MS. I see the benefit in my abilities improving because I exercise and so even though it is by no means a cure, I know it is suppressing the progress of the illness. I am attempting to maintain a plan of exercising daily and probably won't stop even if I need to reduce it with age. I can only gauge changes over a good length of time so I need to put in substantial effort to keep it going before I judge the results. I need to then think back to understand best how, by comparison, my health is lasting and improving with exercise. Even when I get up in the morning, I warm up with some press-ups before anything else. Whatever my plans for the day, I do this as a regular activity, and it is good to get my heart beating and blood flowing so I can come back to a workout when I am ready. If I have at least done this, I can be happy that I am starting on the right foot for the rest of the day.

Being unemployed has given me an opportunity to spend my time working on my health among other things. It is good that this situation has taken place and I am able to move on positively with a new life. It would be wrong to have given up and thought my life was over because of redundancy but I know that when a door shuts, a window opens in life and I think of the door as employment and the window as my new lifestyle. I imagine there are those who, given a serious diagnosis, consider their life to be over and lack the motivation to try to improve the situation. However, when it comes to myself, that was what made me think and act in lots of different ways because I have made use of the extra time I have while it lasts, and I don't want to miss an opportunity. We all have the commodity of time on our hands, and I want to use it in a profitable way and not waste it. It has involved a lot of effort to put together a routine and stay happy but I am proof that it can be done. The important thing is not to give up on your situation and let it pass by; rather, be inventive and creative. Look at what you can do and not what you are unable to do, and this is a positive start. Sure, there are going to be some changes in my abilities but I will still try. See how a chance can rise from every opportunity and work with it so stay alert and if it takes time to start up, don't give up.

Talk to others for inspiration and remember that it may take time and effort to get started, so be prepared for this. I have good and bad days, but this will not phase me because there are so many positive things I can use, like just focusing on the good days, which can help me not to quit. I can meditate when I feel I am struggling, and this refreshes me and finds new and alternative mindsets. I am as hard at work mentally as I am physically, and it is there that lies a solution. I always find a path because it is never a dead end unless you give up and make it one. No surrender.

There are times when I allow myself to have a few beers and eat junk food and I make sure it doesn't happen much or interfere with my main lifestyle because it may develop into a regular occurrence, and I don't want that. It is only a bit of escapism, and this occasion is a time I have carefully considered and allowed as a one-off.

I think about what I eat a lot, and it is mostly a healthy diet with fruit and vegetables, and meat if I want. I am no expert on this subject and can only trust the information available and see how it goes but I am sure I am not far off a good diet because my body is functioning well in that department. It is very occasionally that I don't follow my routine anyway and it will be mainly a special occasion like a party, or A little treat if I've been at the hospital for tests for a long time. I always make up for it though by doing a few extra reps on my shoulders and drinking extra water but not overdoing it. I make sure to eat breakfast and then work out before having a coffee and fruit and then use the remaining time proactively. I drink water at specific times whether I am thirsty or not because I don't want to lose energy and get tired unnecessarily.

Keeping hydrated is so important. Come lunchtime, I do a small workout and eat and then I am free to be meditating and studying for the afternoon. I keep fluid available and I never overdo things and stop my routine right away if it starts to get out of hand. I don't want to injure myself or get dehydrated as that can stop me for maybe a week and I am not happy with this. If I get tired, I will rest, rehydrate then continue when I can. I don't want to lose the routine plan that is in place because it is to help and not hinder me. Success is not built from quitting and the more I do, the better I become at doing it. Just remember, it is no race and so take breaks and relax as needed so it never becomes a big deal.

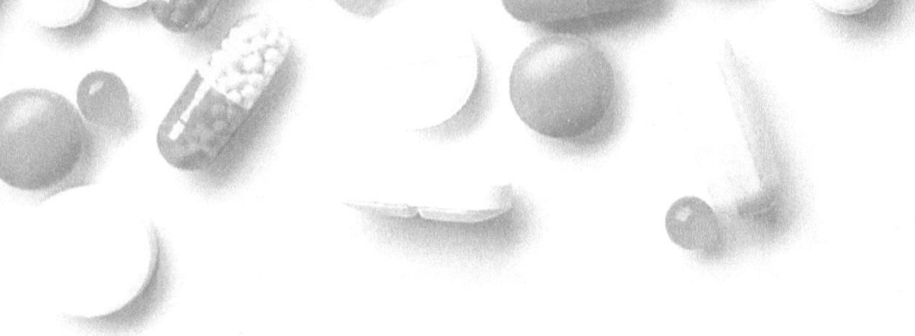

CHAPTER 10

Use all available treatments

Now that I am known by my medical team and have a solid diagnosis, there is so much support available to me. All I need to do is accept the help and support when I need it. Due to my medication, I need a regular blood test which has gone from something I had to do as part of my treatment to so much of a part of life that if I don't have one, I am chasing it. You see, I understand the importance of a blood test to pick up any abnormalities that may occur but also that over time, the test will become less frequent as my body becomes used to the medication. I am now so used to this that I can watch the nurse taking the blood without even thinking about it.

If I have appointments with my neurologist, they will want to see me walk and turn around so they can assess my mobility and see if there is anything that I can be given as an option to improve how I am coping. I have a stick which I use for added stability, especially in warm weather when I need it most. I take the stick with me even if I don't need it, and that way, even if I rely on it because of tiredness, I can still cope with the walking. The main problem the neurologists noticed was that my left foot dropped when I lifted my leg and so they suggest I wear a device to stop that because when my foot was dropping, I trip on changes in the ground. The device fits into my shoe and goes under my foot to support it and then the whole thing is strapped onto my calf and holds my foot up while I walk.

Before going out, there are a few things I need to consider such as distance, temperature and whether there are steps involved. I can use fences and walls, etc., to help with my balance, but I prefer not to as it draws attention to my disability.

I am trying to use as little assistance as I can for as long as I can to preserve my independence, but nothing beats an arm to hold onto.

I'm on immune-suppressing medication that needs to be monitored regularly but that only takes a few appointments a year for some tests, and the time this takes is hardly anything compared to the time I spend travelling and waiting to be seen, so these occasions provide a good time to think and plan. I also have my pulse and blood pressure checked for abnormalities and that test can be taken every quarter. These results are generally good, and I put that down to all the exercise I do which gives me the incentive to keep it up. The fact that regular exercise keeps me healthy is great. Now and then, new and improved treatments and medication become available and if they are suitable, I will change if it makes my life easier, so I am not passive with my life and by no means do I just want to sit back and do nothing, but it is an idea to simplify and improve the treatment if I can. Saying all these things, I must add that the medication that I am on is keeping me stable, and even on the bad days, I can still focus on the good. This can change so it is important to remain positive and it helps if I just get on with life and don't worry too much about that level of treatment and medication only. Getting everything into perspective and arranging my priorities is the most important aspect as this allows me to spend the rest of my time working ion my lifestyle. There may come a day when I need to change my situation permanently, but until then, I am fortunate to be able to afford not to work, giving me the time to pay attention to my health.

When I attend a neurologist appointment, I will be put through some tests and these need to be done in person for obvious reasons, but it is only occasionally so is the least intrusive of all. We discuss any accidents and difficulties I may have encountered with my balance. We also discuss in depth how my everyday life is going – a much more in-depth conversation than is normally available at an ordinary appointment. Obviously, it is easier for the professionals to pick up on any minor changes when I see them face to face, and this includes them watching how I move about. The strength of my grip is also always tested when I demonstrate by squeezing a hand and the general strength of my arms is tested by resistance stretching. I am very good at the strength tests because I exercise my shoulders, but unfortunately, my left foot is weak and drops when I am tired and so that's why I have been fitted with a splint. This splint helps me not to trip on the floor which is going to happen if I can't pick my foot up. I think that the more tired I am, the worse all my problems become.

I have a further test that involves touching my nose and then the neurologist's finger which gets moved at different distances and heights and when my hand shakes it is difficult, but my coordination is okay. Despite my shakes, I can do most things. The general idea is to monitor any changes and so that is why these tests need to be done in person and not over the phone. I understand that during the pandemic, for example, such tests had to be limited, however, it is always better to have a face-to-face appointment rather than over the phone.

My eyesight has been treated at an eye clinic with medication and eventually surgery after a long road of different attempts to control it in various ways. It was not so bad in the beginning, and I started on corrective prisms attached to my spectacles which helped for a while. I then had Botox which involved an injection in the corner of the eye, but it does need to be done regularly and that didn't work out for many reasons. Sometimes the Botox was not available, or the person trained to administer it was away and, in the end, I just gave up on that option.

All the time, I was putting off surgery, however, it turned out that squint surgery was the best move. This was painful though, and not nice for the following week, but it was worth it. It was done under general anaesthetic and it all went well however the real difficulty was with recovery. After the anaesthetic wore off, I was in such pain for a week that at times I couldn't sleep and so I relied on painkillers. I also needed to wear an eye guard when I slept to stop my eye from being touched and I would wake up in the morning with the eye guard stuck on some other part of my body due to my moving in my sleep but fortunately, my eye was okay. There was also a requirement to take eye drops and use specific ointments to aid recovery. I got a lot of the drops down my face because I shake to start with and found that lying on my back when giving myself eyedrops worked best. I was in pain for days and so I took a week off work for a chance to recover. When I went back to work though, lots of people commented on how my eye was facing forward and that the surgery had made a visible difference even if it was just cosmetic. Perhaps one day, I will be free of eye tests, but for now, I still need them as my sight is quite poor. Therefore, I go and see an ophthalmologist every six months and have a thorough eye check-up. First, I get to chat with the optician About how things are going, then it comes to the tests. They check my sight in both eyes using the charts but I'm lucky if I can read a few. They check my colour vision with the book of numbers which is made up of different coloured dots as you go through the pages, and I really struggle with this. The results are all taken, and they are always interested in what medications

I am on at that time because sometimes, they can cause things like glaucoma. It can be a but daunting but also reassuring when you know that they are checking for the least little difference.

When it comes to my daily routine, every part of it has its own level of priority within the mix and none of it will work independently. My medical team has been there to ensure that the medication I am on is the most suitable for me and that everything is in place for me so that all I have to do is take it. I would not dare take risks, especially with my medication.

I have an MRI scan every year to see the extent of damage to my nervous system and whether it has changed. This involves lying on a bench with earphones on and being asked to keep still and then being pushed into the machine. While in the machine, there are loud noises while the scan takes place and sometimes, I am given an injection during the procedure. I know that this is all-important to make sure that the medication is working and that the damage to my nerves is minimalized. The treatment has been tailored to best suit me and I am confident the medical team is doing their best and I don't need to think about it too much. All the tests and scans are coupled with further appointments to monitor me in person which is something I have stayed with. Since the initial problem I had was with my eye, I am keen to see if there is any difference between them and hope that one day, they will offer a solution for the damage to my optic nerves. Although these tests sound like a lot, they are spread across the course of a year leaving me plenty of time for other things. I am thankful for the support, and I feel that given time to adjust, I can get on with it all.

The road I am on is complicated and there is no simple solution, so keeping myself available for treatment is the best thing I can do.

I sometimes need to keep using additional apparatus to get used to it, so it is important not to just give up and think that it is too difficult – give yourself a break and then try again. There is very little excuse for me not to keep all my appointments and use all my equipment because that shows a lack of effort on my behalf. Like with all things in life, taking the easy option is often the most attractive but probably will not benefit you the most, so it is vital that you give it your all when faced with new challenges.

There are some people who need the help and cannot get it, so be grateful for the appointments and care that you are given. It is also a good idea to accept every piece of equipment or care suggestion that can make your life a little easier, after all, they would not supply you with these things if they did not help. MS is a difficult problem to live with and there are times when I struggle but I am up for the challenge and take struggles as par for the course. I am convinced that I stand a better chance if I don't stop trying. From my experience, none of it is nice, just some parts are easier to handle than others. It can take time so accept it because who knows what will happen? Things may improve with some effort involved.

When I had a chance, I spoke with my neurologist about the shaking in my hands so she upped the dose of Gabapentin I take and suggested that wearing weights on my wrists is a possibility to help control this and so I got some half-kilo wrist weights, and they do help control my shakes. I would have never thought of this myself and this goes to show that support is essential. I now consider whom I can talk to as well as what I can do when I develop problems in movement because there is often a solution that I need help to work out. The bonus elementals are, when I am wearing my wrist weights, I can work on my shoulders with some simple exercises and that is right up my street. All in all, I need to use any apparatus I have been given, or it defeats the purpose of having it. Again, trying to be patient while getting used to some items is important and I will not stop. I spend a lot of time making sure everything is comfortable when I use apparatus, from the walking stick being the right length to the orthotics on my foot being a good fit and this, I find, is important so take a bit of time for that. I am fully aware that there is more to dealing with MS than just medication, so I spend a lot of time involved in it. I think it is foolish to let someone else do everything for me because I am not a child. It is important that my routine includes medication, exercise, diet and apparatus for me to benefit the most, and don't forget prayer and meditation. All the different treatment is helping me carry on and not give up, so I am willing to try, and this is being noticed, and For this reason, I am not always being left out of activities due to my condition. I will continue to accept all help or treatment available and even though things may have to be juggled about a bit, I will not give up.

Consider how my medical team views me and how they think about my condition and my work to help them. Am I a patient who just is flippant when it comes to my health and doesn't really try to benefit from the medication and equipment they are supporting me by arranging? Am I a person that doesn't even make sure that I am taking my medication and they have a view of me from this? Or do they see me as a person who cares about themselves so much that they are attending their appointments and spending their free time working hard on their health and want to get on top of MS by taking their medical guidance seriously? Does it interest them to see how I am doing and make them happy to be a part of my endeavours because they can see that I am putting up a strong fight? Will, what I do gain their interest and give them a cause to discuss and think of what is involved in my lifestyle?

Are they going to find themselves asking me about my input? I hope that I can be a source of inspiration in not giving up. I want people to see that they may need to rethink their understanding of illness and the opportunities that they offer to solve what are thought of as unsolvable. If one person finds inspiration, it is a joyous result. This is an opportunity for me to climb what seems to be an insurmountable obstacle and make an example of it. I am using all I can lay my hands on whether it is an easy or difficult job and doing my best through the good and bad. It is a struggle, and I am up for it, like many people are, achieving great things despite adversity. What kind of person do I want to be?

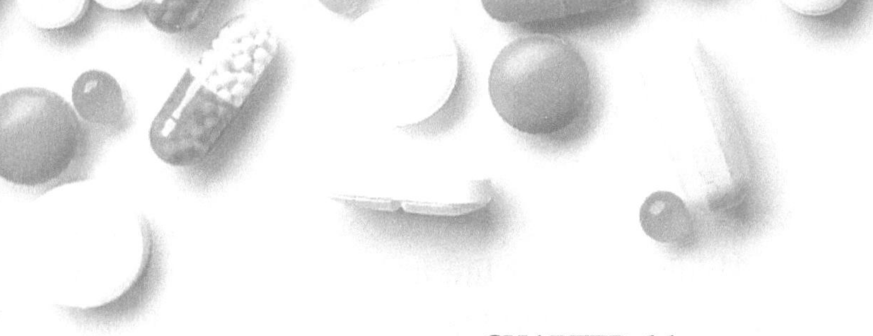

CHAPTER 11

Our heavenly Father is aware of your struggle

I spent my first 20 years uninterested in the Bible and made no attempt at reading or studying it. I always had a Bible and kept it though because I was given one by my godparents when I was christened. I would tell people I was an atheist but that wasn't accurate because an atheist would be someone who had studied scripture and then decided that there is no God. I was just someone who knew nothing about the subject and that was all there was to it. I now understand a true atheist has put time and effort into their belief that there is no God. So, it turns out that there is more effort in being an atheist than just not believing in God. As a pre-Christian, I had no boundaries on how I acted or treated people and a Christian would be able to talk about that conduct. When I decided to read the Bible was when I started to socialize with Christians. At first, as I started reading the Bible, it made no sense and I can understand people who do little else, but as I studied the scripture and kept reading, it eventually started to make logical sense. My life was getting slowly worse and leaving me with no satisfaction before studying scripture and it was this that was making no sense. I was living for entertainment and nothing much else and found days were just going by and the only meaning in life was to enjoy it while it lasted. Even getting married and having a family had no interest to me because without faith, there is nothing but enjoying life while it lasts for them too. There is no guidance to help lead a wholesome life or the prospect of resurrection and a paradise to live in. Thinking about life in a secular way is just bleak but the Bible gives me something to look forward to for everyone who is involved. I was a person that needed this to give me a reason for life which I otherwise see as futile. The faith I will continue to nurture gives real joy and purpose to life. I suppose that I spent enough of my life with a futile outlook and tried to make it work but I need more to give me a reason to truly enjoy a purposeful life and feel that it is not going to just end for us all. The hope I gain even when going through a difficult stretch help's me immensely. I no longer despair.

When I study the Bible, I realise how wonderful it is and how blessed we are that people have even given up their lives to bring it to us all. Those who continue to bring us the Bible have the understanding that it brings hope. I see why the Bible is the best-selling book of all time and that is a good reason to read it even if you don't believe any of it. Spiritually, I am growing in my uprightness, and this is good because I was living a life of possessions and experiences which is all temporary and no more, as I discussed in Chapter 3. As a friend, I speak of the hope that we have and how scripture gives us this and was inspired by Jehovah, our God. Although learning scripture isn't bad at all as an academic exercise, it is so much more enjoyable when it takes over your life and becomes why you are nice and keen on others being enlightened too. I was leading a life based on gaining stuff and the more the merrier, and this was all I thought about and so it was logical to give this belief idea a try. I got involved with a congregation and they helped me understand scripture and how it applies to us. What I am learning is beneficial to understanding my needs are what should be acquired and that is all, so I can forget my wants and be free from desire. It is important that around the world, our needs are met. The understanding and truth are moving me, and this is giving me happiness and joy. I have no more hate or jealousy in my life and don't take risks. My confidence and happiness grow and grow. What I have opened myself up to is wonderful and the gift we all have been given is clearly set out in the Bible. I give time to reading and studying the Bible and prayer because I am studying Christianity and dedicating myself to Jehovah. I spend time with fellow Christians and live a life in a less fleshly way which, surprisingly, is less stressful. I no longer worry about how much and what other people have and only what I have. I don't care who is most successful or has the most important position at work. I am clothing myself in a Christian personality because it is the truth and I finally understand this. I guess you could liken my life, up until I found spirituality, to just wandering aimlessly. When my faith became real to me, I finally saw that there is more to life than what I could see and touch, like the importance of love and peace.

I became a Christian in my late twenties thanks to my father who is a bit spiritual, and as our relationship grew, he thought it would benefit if I got involved in a church of some sort by attending an Alpha course. Everything happened about the time I was diagnosed with MS. I became a Christian and it was a matter of keeping involved and not letting my health concerns get in the way because my faith is permanent which is more than I can say about some relationships with people. I didn't have time for Jehovah until my thirties and had spent my time enjoying myself, which I still do but now not in an unclean way thanks to Christianity, like when I would spend my spare time overeating and drinking too much alcohol. I am learning the value of the Bible and how I benefit from its advice on my health, like self-control, among other things. The whole arrangement suits me together with my lifestyle and without it, I don't know what state I would be in because of my health requirements. Above everything, I learn that our heavenly Father wants the best for us and will always be with us even in death. I don't think anyone can offer us the same commitment God can. I am studying the scripture and getting guidance so that I can understand the big picture. By this, I mean as much as I can about life, the universe, and everything. The gift our heavenly Father has given us is breath-taking and something I will be indefinitely trying to repay. I pray and give Jehovah's worship daily to show my thanks and associate with fellow believers when I can. There are lots of things that are beneficial to all who are good Christians because I know that there is more than just knowing right; I am trying to act this way too. It is like knowing the correct thing to do is not enough and I need to also *do* what is correct. I am not perfect and only time and dedication are what is needed if I can get close, so it is important to keep with it and not think I have done enough and stop. Over time, I am behaving more in line with Christians which gives me hope beyond the world and a chance to live in paradise. There is a God, and all the evidence is there if you don't get misled by Satan.

Throughout the Bible are pearls of wisdom to help even when I feel I am at my lowest and most at risk of attack from Satan leaving me with depression. I am looking at the Bible and can't fault it as I maybe did before. It has proven itself but it has taken me some time to get here. The Bible is all working together in concordance even though it was put together by many different books and authors and written over many years. As I thought of myself as an unbeliever, I had many disagreements over faith and now I know that I wasn't going anywhere, and I lacked the spirit needed to persevere. I thought all this, and I hadn't even read any of the Bible which was just silly. How can I talk about a film, for example, without watching it myself? Sure, there are always reviews available, but they are not my opinion and someone else has given them. It is like thinking I know about somebody's health without doing any research and then talking to them which a doctor would at least do. Now I understand that I can have dedication always because it is there for anyone who works at it and will always be. My life has found new meaning, and I will never move on without my belief and how I now read about it daily to keep me from being a nihilist. I have chosen a direction that I will stay with, and I am healthier and happier, and people can see this in me and so there is evidence of its benefit. I endeavour to pray every day to do more than just know the way so that I may walk in the way which is righteous and right in the Bible for us all to learn. I need the spirit I gain from prayer to give me wisdom and courage in my life. I often wonder what Jehovah is doing, fixing, and moving that I don't even know about and imagine how I probably won't understand.

I can say that twenty years ago, I was spiritually dead with a pointless life and had settled into it and now I have faith in Jehovah, I am happy and a changed man. I was dead to sin, and this is what I see in retrospect, and I only know this with the availability of the Bible and learning to act in accordance with its teachings. The more I read, the more the Bible proves itself with prophecy that has come true historically as proof of its truth. Although I thought I was living a real life, it was just futile and led me to exist and nothing else. When I think about the endowment on offer from our heavenly Father that I was missing out on, I want to share what I now know with others because I want them to not miss out on benefits too. I wish I had been brought up with time spent in faith instead of what society offered – I would have found this way better all round. At the school I attended, there were prayers during assembly but that was about it and any Bible-based education wasn't taken seriously. At home, there was no prayer or Bible study overseen by my family and I would have seen the benefit of spending time together once a week for this. I think a family needs to spend time together.

Reading the Bible left me with a lot of questions, and this is what keeps me interested and going back to read again and find understanding and search for clarity. It would have been easy to say to myself that it makes no sense and put it away and forget about it and this is indeed what I did for many years. However there came a time when I kept on studying and re-reading the Bible and this gave me a good understanding of Jehovah and his son Jesus and their qualities, so, over time, my interest is growing. This is how I can build a relationship with them and that is important to me now. Reading and meditating on the Bible is how I am going to spend some time each day now. I am building a relationship that I need to help me follow the righteous life which is essential for a Christian. I have found people who do the same and I am not alone in my direction so feel I have joined a family of which I have now become a part, a family whom I see every week and talk with. I have not replaced my brother and father and hope they understand that I have just grown into friends and people I can turn to. The more I learn and understand, the greater my confidence that it is the truth and that all things will be set straight in time. Therefore, I urge people to read the Bible and find a Bible-based organization to get involved with while they can. My friends and family spend less and less time with me because they have their own commitments, and I am happy for them. My growth as a Christian is a joyous thing for me and I think it will help me not feel alone. I walk with Christians, something we can all do, and this is the perfect time to talk and consider the good news as in the gospels. We spend time worshipping and reading Jehovah's word in the Bible together at weekly meetings which enables us all to understand better as well as talk about our experiences and struggles with each other and gain support.

There will be time to forget about the temporary and fast and give thanks for the gift of the eternal for those who want to. In Matthew, Jesus said, "I am the way, the truth, the life". He didn't say 'I am one of the ways of truth and you can make a choice about it' but what Jesus said is a fact and he is the only way. As it teaches in Matthew 24:13: "But the one who has endured to the end will be saved". Basically, this means don't give up, so I keep faithfully praying for wisdom and the strength to carry my burden. Quite simply, through Jesus, we can approach Jehovah in prayer, and we should never stop doing so because it may be our last chance. I am keen to obey and serve the sovereign heavenly father and I don't have a problem with this because there is no problem with this, and I accept people disagree and that is their choice, and all I want to do is ensure I am living with faith. If nonbelievers talk to me, I will be interested in their views and beliefs and share mine. I have self-discipline and the understanding to see what will come will come is better than other options. So, I read and study the Bible daily and make sure I have the time to do so which may mean a small sacrifice that is nothing to worry about to me. Walking with believers is a wonderful opportunity to show my devotion and share experiences and friendships. Jehovah has opened a door that nobody can shut.

Study and learn from Jesus and Christians and find that you will adjust your behaviour to serve and help to shepherd others even when you find it hard going and don't feel the benefits that the Almighty heavenly Father's followers feel. We are imperfect humans and there are going to be hard times that will test a person's faith, so it is important to keep the faith and there is always a chance to pray for a petition. Prayer is always available, and you don't need an appointment, only give it some thought first, and Jehovah is the hearer of prayers. If you need help, pray in your time of need, and remember you are not alone and there are fellow followers to talk with who can offer to show support and guidance also. I think many people fear being ridiculed and targeted for their beliefs and shut themselves away when they need to be strong and open, have courage and show love and not hate or fear. In the Bible, there are accounts of people who maintained their faith during times of distress when their friends abandoned them. I know how to study and learn because I have spent years on qualifications that have cost lots of money and time so studying was part of the process and something I could draw on at times. All that time, there was a Bible and Christian organization available at no cost and I should have made use of it sooner but that was just a thought and doesn't really matter now I am involved and gaining faith. Sure, I have been on the wrong path, but it is never too late to change and turn back to the right way and be on the right path which is very rewarding no matter where you come from. Take the apostle Paul, for example, and the life he led before he found Jesus on the road to Damascus and then changed. In life, I hear of those involved in crime and drugs who change. I now make time to maintain a Christian life and enjoy a community of believers. I get people reminding me of my past sometimes and with my understanding, I see if there is an opportunity there to talk about where I am now heading and teach the gospel including how I have changed. At times like these, it is important to listen and think about what I say and try to engage with people and show friendship. The goal is to maintain peace and that is very important in a happy life. This is the truth that we lost thanks to desires.

Remember to praise God and don't be afraid to stand up for what you believe in, even if it means standing alone. You may feel you are alone, however, Jehovah, our God will be with you always and you are never alone. I don't care what people think anymore because I only care what Jehovah thinks. Generally, there is a misleading and lying trait that Satan has always been using to gain certain people's thoughts and turn their beliefs against Christians. I know from my pre-Christian days what arguments I would use against believers. I look to the Bible for understanding and guidance nowadays. As far as the Bible goes, I inherited MS and Jehovah has put in place salvation for us. This is because of the original sin and how it is passed down through the generations. This belief gives me comfort on this and many things that have been wrong in the world. Please understand I do have belief in how paradise was lost. When the hand of God is on your life, nobody can stop you from being blessed. Feel the truth in life and turn away from all the lies. I know soon, God's Kingdom, or heavenly government, will intervene in earth's affairs. (Daniel 2:44) That government will eliminate the cause of human suffering and ensure that God's will is done on the earth.—Matthew 6:9, 10.

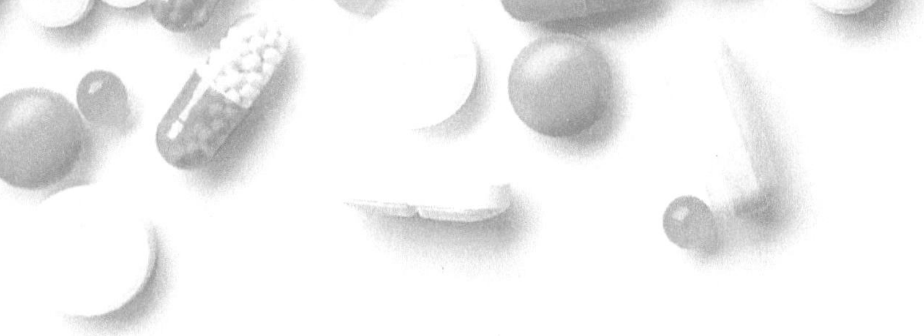

CHAPTER 12

Keep going with all that you can

To start with, you must tell yourself, "no matter how hard it gets, I am going to make it work". Once I had a routine in place, then I laid down a course to follow it and this will stay in place and not get replaced or changed and is simply achieved each day. I am convinced this routine must be kept up. It may increase or decrease over time, but the basic structure is solid and adhered to. The work is not finished; I may think it is, but it isn't. In fact, it has just begun. Once a routine is laid down, it is important to follow it up and the reward will be improved health. Quite simply, I am doing the exercises and hydrating myself a lot, and in the new lifestyle, there is a fundamental change in my existence. This means that the work will not finish and there will always be more to do, and this is something that needs to be accepted. There will be no time when I can think I have done enough and can finish. I understand that it all starts with me from the ground up and so I am always available to do what is right for my health and look after myself for the future throughout the days. Above my own responsibilities are the work of medical experts to ensure I have my medical needs met as far as medication and monitoring how my condition goes and that really doesn't take too much of my time and continues as well. The medical side of things is ongoing and will not stop for me either but is not as involved as my exercising because exercising, eating, and hydrating take up most of my time. Then, above it all, I trust in our heavenly Father and keep faith in both my understanding and behaviour and give it time for prayer and meditation always.

I will try and keep my new lifestyle, which focuses on healthy living through diet and exercise, in place for all my days. I am now eating mainly vegetables, I put extra virgin olive oil on a lot of what I am eating, and drink loads of fluids as part of my diet, so I keep this all up. Things do tend to fall into place so that it seems I have time for it all. My purpose has changed from getting up and going to work five days a week and I am now less focused on possessions and more on my health which sounds very involved, but I do have time to spare, so I don't need to worry if I stop to watch a film or listen to music. I am now very busy in my new life and don't have too much free time left and this makes me feel happy. I can always find things to do even if the medical treatment is out of my hands but needs to take place and so I fit things around it which is everything else and involves most of the time. My lifestyle may have needed to change, and I need to be awake and aware of this and observe it so I can do what I need to maintain a healthy routine. It is all like a full-time job and I only really take Sunday off to attend worship. I don't want to overdo it, though, and especially in the summer when it becomes more difficult due to the temperature and how it affects my energy. Still, where there is a problem, there is a solution and I take cold showers to help with this because the important thing is to keep going and so that is what I do, keep going. There are times when it is a real mental effort to battle on, so I need to get some help from Jehovah in prayer to keep me strong. Who knows where this is all going? We can only wait and see...

The items I need to keep in control of are to be part of my life and it is important not to burn the steps. So, I keep a note of them as follows:

Continuously build a routine of activities

1. It is important to keep on top of treatment and medication. There are side effects and times you will need to dig deep and maintain everything prescribed.

2. Diet is important, and you must eat and drink well, and this all needs to be healthy.

3. Exercise whatever your condition and keep it up so make changes if necessary.

4. Emotional health is important so keep an outlook toward peace and harmony and meditate on this.

5. Faith is going to help find strength and hope in a broken world.

These items are my framework for surviving MS, and I keep them in mind every day and will work to not forget them by regularly doing them. The framework has given me the means to create a routine that takes me into a survival way of life and without this framework, I may forget and miss out activities that I do. When I take all things into consideration, it is a package of measures that I can use in any situation in which I find myself. Things happen in life and even if I lose my way and find myself lost because of unexpected occurrences, this list will help me to get back on course and rebuild a routine. Together with my chart of daily activities, I have the tools needed to recreate a routine if necessary and without all the time I originally spent on starting one from scratch. This is how I keep going and it is tremendously useful. It doesn't matter what life throws at me; I am prepared to put what I need in place to have a solution. The health issue can be big and needs a routine that takes a lot of our time to follow, like mine, or maybe a less complex one just to maintain good health. In whatever eventuality, be up for this work.

It is important to set up some basics on how to conduct yourself if you need to improve anything and I have used my experiences and mistakes to do this. You see, I am not perfect, but I have taken the potential, which is what I have in me, and that is how I continue through everything and don't quit. The understanding is that I can find an answer to the reason I get up in the morning and start my routine. What is needed is to focus on a goal and have the dedication to aim for it even if you miss ... just don't give up. If I miss the goal, I will keep trying and maybe I will get successful. It really is worth the effort. Even with success, I want to perfect the aim and that will involve practice and enjoyment because what I am doing needs to become something permanent if possible. The whole idea is key, or I will probably give up and become complacent which will not help my situation. The drive that I gain from setting up a framework that I use stops me from emotionally sitting back and not just looking at the work that needs to be done and procrastinating over it. It has all been developed through stages and has grown into something I am happy to maintain. I have kept one eye on overcoming adversity and accepting it as part of life while doing something about it in the process. It is understandable to think I am achieving nothing because it is a slow process, and I need to think way back to the start so this gives me an idea of how far I have come and that is motivating me to see how much further I can get from here on in. Thinking like this is the only way to gauge the size of a job like this one. Therefore, I am finding any way I can to give reason for my activities and these reasons may need to change over time to offer ongoing encouragement. Why not try using several reasons, and then, if one does not do it, think of another one to switch to? I need to take those times of difficulty and those times of ease together because they are changes in one activity. Maybe keep a diary or something to refer to and help find out how you deal with difficulties as and when you faced them. Always congratulate yourself on how well you are doing and that whatever you have done is a good achievement so you will keep pushing further. Tell yourself well done even when you get up. I think the hardest thing is motivating myself but the longer I spend on anything, the more it becomes a part of life.

I wish I could say that if you stick with a routine for a month or a year, that should be enough to solve any problems, but I cannot so just congratulate yourself when and where you can. Unfortunately, I need to make time to stick with a routine for the rest of my life and there is no doubt that I can stop with wishful thinking and excuses, but I won't because the stakes are too high for me. To be honest, I can't think too far into the future anyway, so I take it a day at a time, and that way I am making sure the basics are covered and the whole idea of time is not too overpowering. Things change and I need to be versatile and adapt my routine to meet my needs, but the basics always remain in place now. I will not stop meeting my needs and that means I will not stop a routine because I don't think it's doing anything. You see, my routine is an important part of my life like eating or breathing and therefore essential. There are times I need to think about what I may have missed and that is okay because reflecting on how I am getting on reminds me to continue. Sometimes I see a cup of coffee that I haven't drunk and need to put that right and drink it. I will find some spare time and put things right if I think of anything I need to do and have missed it. Just like the medication, I may think the routine is not working, but I will remain strong and trust it to be working in the background. The important thing is I don't give up based on the way I feel about life at any time because when I get started, it will change my feelings from negative to positive again. What I am trying to maintain is way above feelings, and I know this. Survival is the purpose and if I am going to survive, I must consider that what I do is the best way for me to behave. That is why your routine is something you must persist in to get any results, so don't give up – find your own potential.

I have written this to help me to remember everything I am doing to survive MS and it was only going to be a testimony at the start, so I can't have given up on that. Keep going and realize that it takes time and persistence and eventually things happen. Out of an acorn, a mighty oak can grow - I guess what I am saying is to stick with the task and let it grow as a tree does. I don't see dead ends but instead, look for opportunities to solve the puzzles and this is good for the mind. It is a case of taking a problem and finding a solution in whatever form it takes. Everything has a solution to improve productivity or repurpose what is there. I sometimes find there are things I need to use faith to move on with because they are more than I can contemplate. I never think I don't have time or it's too difficult because that is not the way to think. The way to think is there is a large mountain in the way, and I am going to get through, around, or over it. Some things involve stopping and remembering that I might need to change my approach to the problem to find a solution because I wasn't expecting that, so I need to change my understanding. I may need to write it down and come back to it at another time or risk letting it stop proceedings as normal because some exercise and a coffee break are needed sometimes and then work on the problems can restart. Where there is hope, there is a way.

This much I do know - MS will not stop, and it will not take a rest or a holiday and so I must not stop and take a rest from my routine either. I need to deal with this like for like. If I let MS get out of control, and it can if you let it, I am risking permanent problems with my health, and everything will become more difficult so do I want this to happen? I think it is possible to keep MS stable and have an okay life. Things are already hard enough, and I don't want them to get worse and have the added emotional problem bashing around my head that I could have done something. I can liken MS activity to time and how time will continue to pass irrespective of whether it is watched or not. There are different severities of most illnesses and so it is always important to keep at work on my simultaneous efforts that will complement the medical treatment. I can stop acknowledging the time and that will not stop it from passing so I keep going and accept that time is just relative. The only effect is on me not being up to date with my planned routine and everything else and so it has its use. It is possible that I am always going to be running uphill and, by that, I mean finding it hard going. So, keep up to date with coping with MS and how the best methods may have changed, and do as much as possible even if it is hard going because if not it will only become harder, so the choice is to do or not to do. To do this is going to need dedication and giving things a chance to improve, so I ask myself if this is what is wanted or not. Time will need to be put aside to deal with MS and this means making sacrifices. Use your time wisely and make sure the important things are done. Take medication and exercise, for if you take a break and stop, you are at risk of MS causing more damage to your health or even getting comfortable and comfortable does not lead to success. Success is challenging work and not comfortable living. Don't sit around waiting for a cure because who can say how long that will take? It is now you need to work against the effects of MS on your nervous system and sitting around is not going to achieve anything. Some things take too much time to act out. Therefore, in the meantime, keep going.

The message here is to do it and do your best. I give myself carte blanche in the life I pursue and how hard the level I am on gets because I have been doing it for decades. I know full well the problem I am taking on and I am very serious when I say to someone that I am working on a process to deal with it. The average person can see what I am achieving if they meet me. This boils down to what you can do and while you are alive, you are capable of more than you realize because you are putting in an effort that will turn into more capability within yourself over time. I do not just say this to people, but it is what I live. Basically, I am practising what I preach every day and it is definitely a help. Do not give this a bit of a go without dedication to a purpose and reaching for this. What I do is what I can and as much as I can and that is the idea because if it is kept up, then it will change the body and be amplified by time. The basic idea is to continue with this purpose if you want to achieve anything, and the longer the better. The body will become stronger and fitter and help cope with the problems it has so remember that there is more to think about than what you want to achieve - you need to think about the process too. It is no lie that it takes effort and lots of it, so the mind must adapt to think along these lines. Without the desire to do this, it is going to become pointless and options to get out of exercising something will become powerful and are going to take control. It is foolish to give up because you will become better at what you do if you keep doing your best. We all start at a point and need to practice if we want to improve. Set a routine up and do your best to maintain it and let the medication do what it does so that together, it all makes a difference. There is no time I consider that I have tried it and it hasn't worked so instead, I consider it is still working and hasn't finished working and needs to continue. These things are in our control and we mustn't waste this opportunity. Use mind over matter.

Do not compare yourself to others. No one can play your role better than you so all you can do is learn from others and cherry-pick what is useful to you. The length of time you have been at work on a system is going to show in your abilities and comparing one person with another might be a case of comparing heaps of experience with a person with little experience and is like comparing a professional with an amateur. This is not a competition so we are all finding how we need to survive in our way, and even if there are similarities, we are going to need to find our unique way and keep going. It is not the easiest for me to type but I am able to, in my way, get on with it and the more I do, the more I can. I am always struggling with my right hand, which shakes, but I have not let that stop me. I think it just means I am different from others or the normal style, and I don't care. Other people should focus on what I can achieve and not what I need to do differently to overcome my differences. So what if I am different? I am not going to hide away and ghost everyone; just some maybe. I am visually impaired or whatever the accepted terminology for it is and that is the last thing to consider so I first consider what I can do to help me to carry on, such as using large print. Deep breathing seems to help me stay calm and get on through work when I get frustrated. I am still going after decades of self-belief and so I must be doing something right. I am thankful for the purpose I have in life and can be happy with keeping active in my body and thoughts because there is more to benefit from this way. I am looking to the future and not the past. I have given myself a new direction and, as they say, a door may close, but a window will open. Therefore, keep finding new options and let go of the past because it is beneficial this way. It is important to me to have a way to go and targets to reach and so I am up to changing myself and my career when necessary to achieve exciting new things. I am in a situation where change is necessary, and it is important to work on changes because of that and not because I feel like it. The alternative would leave me lost and without hope with monsters in my head. If there are times I am lost and aimlessly doing nothing, then I can pick up the Bible and read, or listen to scripture online if that is easier, and it is a source of encouragement to see what Joseph, for example, went through and he always did his best. I am enduring the routine I am following so there are many things going on in my life to occupy me. Hopefully, I can keep going. Being occupied will keep me from bad and pointless activities when I should be doing my best to stick with an important routine. I will keep going and do my best.

Don't stop until you have no option and even then, look for new opportunities and new ways to continue. Basically, if I stop, I try to keep it for as short a time as possible. If you were in a job, you would have a line of tasks needing to be done during the day, so keep it the same with your routine. I will be working unpaid even if I dislike being on benefits and always want to support myself. I am in charge and will do what is needed to run this company that is me and want it to improve and not go out of business. It is important to have a healthy view of life and live it. I can always tailor my routine if I need to because this is what it takes sometimes to continue successfully. The main point is to look to achieve something and not quit and stop. If I put time aside to follow my routine, I have made the first step and must continue to take steps and use the time to do this work. I am unable to do what I want and that's useable. So mentally, the struggles need me to work on them and I want the work so the struggles will pass, therefore, I have gained a raison d'être. It is a mission to keep going and I see where I want to be so I can set a course for it. Sure, it is not always the easiest endeavour, and I may need to socially sacrifice because I need to work on my health first, so any sacrifice is for the best. I know full well my limitations and they are the rules that must not break me and guide me instead because I can try to decrease them. I find that there are plenty of people to talk to and explain this to even if they continue not to fully realise my limitations because, for example, I don't like the heat and I am repeatedly invited out when it's hot. There is work to be done both on my tolerance of heat and my way of explaining this issue to someone. My neighbours and people I meet are a few who mean well, and I don't mind trying to explain these things to them more than once because it is good practice for me. Sure, my times no longer fit in with everybody else's but there is always an opportunity to talk to someone new and find common ground. So, the old ways I used to socialise have changed and I have changed to accommodate this and maybe the social life I was leading was bad anyway. I now think of my medical team as my work colleagues who give me the work I need to put in for my health. For the main part of this, I am doing my work and only occasionally need some help. The people who have faith in the Bible are now my friends, and so on.

If you are struggling, I sincerely hope you can gain encouragement from me and understand that the requirements are nothing to fear and just a lot of hard work. Satan will use fear to mislead, however, love will beat that and so, over time, I have started to love this work and keep doing my best. The work I undertake has become part of who I am. The life I lead is not easy and sometimes I question it with my hand on my heart and can't see enjoyment through it all, but not all the time because there are good times too. I think I probably was never satisfied as an employee either, so this gives me relief for a while because it is never boring working for myself and makes me feel I am accomplishing something important for me. I don't expect my situation will stay the same, but in one way or another, I am feeling good about My way of living because I love what I am doing to help it. I understand that I have changed and need to deal with the fact, or I risk going mad. It takes time and the right attitude to survive MS and I am always at work on it, so I get all the doubts going and feel I am letting many people down, but I don't worry about what people think as much as what Jehovah God thinks. Any negative thoughts and doubts that are in my head can be easily evicted by me. I wish to thank all those who have, until now, and will in the future, helped me to use my drive and struggle through situations. This is how I carry on with doubts and fear and tiredness. It is all in the mind and will need maintenance as well to stay positive. Sometimes I am going to struggle to maintain my discipline, and this happens from time to time and it's okay to struggle, just don't quit. There will be obstacles that I can't get past and insurmountable problems like not liking the heat. This rules out going outside a lot during the summer but it doesn't stop me from working on it. Also, there are always places that are not outside that I can still go to. I never do anything that puts my health at risk anymore and at the least, I drink water and eat bread.

See, I am putting everything together to complete a routine that does the best, and this is important. I am taking everything into account and taking it as a life choice to replace a life I was in that I felt was pointless because of my health changing and have found an opportunity and run with it. It has taken time and effort to get into a sufficient routine. I have decided to take my life forward in a new direction which will hopefully lead me through difficulties caused by MS and give me a life that is good. There need to be the necessary adjustments to accommodate, and this may slow me down. I do everything from taking medication to exercising and being spiritually awake. Stopping is not an option.

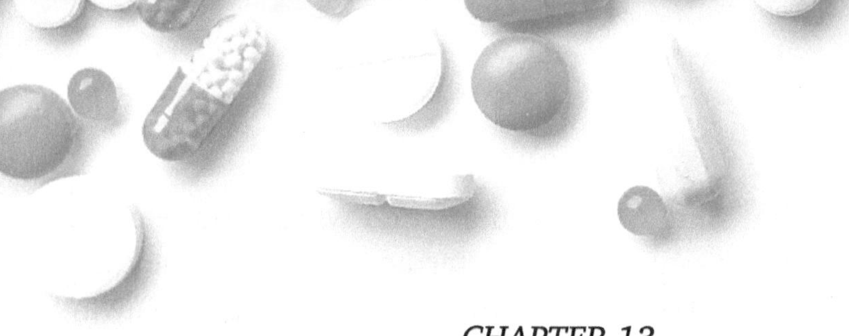

<h1 style="text-align:center">CHAPTER 13</h1>

The new normal has arrived

I am living a new life that includes all the things I have gone over and put in place. The key is to understand that I am doing everything for a good reason and that is to improve my life with MS. If I keep hold of this thought, then I am going to be able to keep my new life all up. The only way I can see it working is if I don't stop and that is why it is an important new lifestyle and a new normal. You see, the interesting thing to understand is it is a variety of things that I am doing, and I don't really know how much they will achieve. My best hope is not to stop MS but to survive MS. I see the difficulties all the time when I am in the company of fellow sufferers and we all want to get better and the only difference is everyone seems to want to achieve this objective in a different way. We are all trying to continue as best as we can, and this is important to keep the mind in a good place. Whether people accept they need to do something or accept that they can wait for the result to happen unchallenged, it is a new normal way to think. Let's be serious and do something other than just think. I am sure that there are some actions that need to be part of life and the important word here is actions. I know that I am better off with a bit of exercise in life and we all should exercise even if it is just a ten-minute walk every day. So, we all have a job to do to keep a healthy body and mind if we want to enjoy life. Understanding what we need in our lives is the start of building a sensible routine that suits where you are and where you want to get. Don't worry if you struggle to get started because, as they say, Rome wasn't built in a day. The best thing we can do is chip away at tasks when we can.

I have put everything in order so then I am free to achieve the items that come up at the top of my routine. This includes any eye tests or trips out to see friends for a meal. I try to be positive and think that there is a blessing coming and am always thankful when good things happen. When things change, it is time to make an amendment that fits safely into the plan, but if things get out of hand, remember to relax because mistakes are not welcome but panicking is not helpful. This may be a temporary stage anyway, and honestly, I can only think of everything this way if I want to keep calm. Through tears and pain on this planet, I have been able to learn how to live in concordance with what has become my new normality. When I am working, there will come a time when I hit a figurative brick wall and this can be dangerous if I don't stop for a break. Too many times I have carried on without a care in the world and had an accident. The condition means I must now be aware of the warning signs of fatigue even before they take effect. This existence needs special understanding from me. I must no longer pass a point that I know full well from experience is dangerous. I have learned these lessons and put them into practice. My life has a fair number of dos and don'ts in it and I count myself lucky that situations I have been in haven't got out of hand. I feel fear and use this feeling. Yes, I can be scared of doing things before I do them, and this is a sign that I should stop and not do said things.

I have come to understand that the time I have on my hands is the best opportunity to do something and that is the point I have in mind. My activities potentially give me hope to at least remain stable and not deteriorate. I am sure the way to move forward is to keep using everything I can reasonably do to achieve this. This is the way I have convinced myself that I must continue and, no matter what happens, I am giving it a good attempt to live with my condition. I am happy that my routine is helping me because it is one I have tailored to my needs and will maintain. The things I am doing have become my life and my new life's work. There are many things to which I have had to become accustomed and this is important. There is no point in maintaining a routine only when I can be bothered. What I do is definitely what I can to keep busy and that is the essence. I found it a real challenge to set up a new life and turn my back on the old one. It takes dedication and a desire that is strong enough to fulfil everything needed. Only when I had arranged the basic requirements was I able to let go of how I used to live fully and completely re-invent myself. I knew it was going to be a big undertaking and I just took it a day at a time and tried to keep going. Mentally, it is important that I prioritise my activities and that means I can't do everything and so I accept this. If I, for example, tell a person that they should start by eating food and drinking water regularly, then it is up to that person to do this and that is where they need to fuel their own behaviour in doing this. They need to persist if they want to benefit totally but it may take some time to happen, so think the sooner the better and get on with it. Once a new system is in place, it will take root and grow.

I have worked through trial and error to find a set of activities to overcome the difficulties I suffer from and simultaneously put my old normal behind me. When I look back over this process, it is something that has happened bit by bit and was never my intention at the start. In order to gain a new normal, I have been through a process of mutation and not given in until I reached my target. I am only feeling satisfaction because I have got this far despite all the obstacles. The goal is always changing and I must be prepared to do the same. The new normal is a reinvention of a life that continues to survive because I am willing to put in the effort required. The way forward is to assess what I need to do to remain as healthy as possible and be able to do what I can. If there are situations that are testing me to the edge of my abilities, it is time to evaluate them. I now have some level of experience and success that acts as self-motivation. In one way or another, there is plenty to be proud of that I am still making an effort and finding success in areas that may have been easy to write off instead. The reason I am still going is the belief that nothing is impossible. Nothing is out of reach and if I can just find a way then I can reach any target. I may no longer be able to run but I can still walk and even if it takes longer, it is still going to get me there. As a rule, I am going for the distance and that is the way with MS or many other illnesses.

Dealing with problems like when I spend too much time on my feet is an opportunity to learn the best way to act. Sometimes I have trouble getting up after being sat down too long and so my condition is complicated. I don't always understand the best actions and sometimes get them wrong, but I try to understand that sometimes I will have difficulties and there isn't much I can do about that. I am in a life where I know how to act most of the time though and that goes enough for now. All I do and achieve in my life to become able to cope with my illness is the life I have built and I am living in it. The new life is serving me better than where my life was heading, and it needed to be rearranged if I was going to stand a chance. The steps I take are based on lots of experience and advice. There is always a person who thinks there is no hope and I disagree, so don't waste time trying to prove them wrong and instead, find people who are open to the idea of hope. The way forward is to build a routine and stick with it as a new normal. I understand if a person has spent decades in a life they are used to, they may find it difficult to see that they can't continue in that way and must start over in a new life and that is why I suggest they take it a day at a time. I would struggle to take it all in at once and so don't overthink it because it is a scary prospect. Find a way to motivate yourself to move on with life. Find a positive viewpoint and hold on to that.

The idea is to be set in a routine and so it is like a daily occurrence along with everything I do as part of a normal life. There needs to be a firm decision made. Blending everything I needed to mould myself into a new cycle took time. I need to know what I am doing throughout each day. From dawn to dusk I am busy, and it is like I have a job to do which pays me in improved health. My health must come in front of money and fame. My health must be worth the effort and any sacrifice to pursue pleasure. I will make my health a high priority. I hope for the best and do what I can. I have focused on me for a reason – my best health.